ANGELINE POMPEI

The Ultimate Anti-Aging Guide

Get Angeline's 3D Anti-Aging Formula And Maintain Your Youth

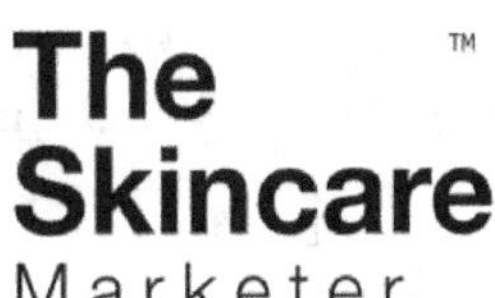

First published by Angeline The Skincare Marketer Inc. 2022

The recommendations in this book and my guidelines for Angeline's 3D Anti-Aging Formula™are completely based on my experience. I, Angeline Pompei and/or Angeline The Skincare Marketer Inc., have not performed any clinical studies and cannot validate any of my claims with hard, factual data aside from the studies and references cited at the end of this book. Before starting any treatment plan, please consult your treating physician or practitioner for safety. Your treatment center, is ultimately responsible for the outcome of your treatments and you should therefore ensure they are aware of your complete medical background. This includes any medications you are taking or have taken over the years before moving forward with any treatment plan. Many medications can make you light/photo sensitive, and many auto-immune diseases may not make you a suitable candidate for many treatments. Hormones also have a huge impact, on your skin health. If you suspect you may have a hormonal imbalance, see your doctor. Certain laser treatments will likely not improve your skin if the root cause is internal. You want to ensure that any health condition you have or have had, are not a contra-indication for any specific treatment. Certain exfoliation treatments may irritate aged skin. Those with dermatitis of other skin issues may not be candidates for certain treatments. Radiofrequency or electricity based treatments (RF) are not suitable for with pacemakers. Those with epilepsy should not be undergoing any laser or light treatments. Cancer patients must also consult their treating physicians prior to starting any treatment plan and should be cancer free for a certain period of time before starting any laser or light procedures. Those who are pregnant should not be performing any cosmetic treatments. Please make sure you disclose your full medical history to your treating physician or practitioner prior to starting any treatment plan. This book serves as a guide only for educational purposes. It is not an absolute solution to anti-aging and the suggestions or claims I, Angeline Pompei or Angeline The Skincare Marketer Inc., make are not absolute recommendations for anti-aging or any cosmetic corrective treatments. Results also vary based on individual lifestyle and ethnicity. If you decide to follow my 3D Anti-Aging Formula™ it is at your own risk and I, Angeline Pompei and/or Angeline The Skincare Marketer Inc.are not liable for any skin or health outcomes that may result from following my guidelines or recommendations. Although you already made the decision to purchase this book, if you decide to proceed with reading this book, it is at your own risk.

First edition

This book was professionally typeset on Reedsy.
Find out more at reedsy.com

Contents

Preface

This book encompasses my almost 20 years of experience in the cosmetic laser industry. My name is Angeline Pompei. I was an Aerospace Engineer who took the risk of quitting my professional career in order to pursue a business opportunity in the cosmetic laser industry. Anti-aging or staying youthful is not a new trend. From the age of the pyramids, we have been trying to stay looking younger longer. Due to my physics background in combination with my aesthetics diploma, I was naturally drawn to the physics of cosmetic treatments.

This book will hopefully educate you on different types of cosmetic and laser treatments for anti-aging and give you some background on the skin. I finish with my 3D Anti-Aging Formula and by describing my own skincare routine to maintain my youth in my 40's. I do believe we should all take care of our skin, from the inside-out and outside-in, however I also believe we should maintain a healthy attitude towards cosmetic treatments. Skincare is healthcare so we need to find a healthy balance between vanity, confidence and healthcare for our physical and mental health. At the end, you can create your own general treatment plan with my 3D Anti-Aging Formula™!

The purpose of this book is for educational purposes. This book is not a replacement for a proper, in clinic consultation and skin assessment.

1

Introduction

Prevention is always better than correction. Once one experiences skin laxity, lines and/or wrinkles, it takes a lot more time, energy (literally laser energy) and money to correct the skin. From my experience, the treatments I cover in this book are optimal for anti-aging. My approach to anti-aging is 3-dimensional. This book starts off with a bit of skin biology and I conclude this book with my 3D Anti-Aging Formula which you can use as a guide if you wish.

If you are interested in learning about how to correct different skin concerns, look for my book "The Ultimate Skin Correction Guide."

This book hopefully gives you a better foundational understanding and explanation of what anti-aging treatments are, and how they work. Cosmetic treatments are elective procedures however, we need to remember that they are still medical procedures and medical devices.

This book is not a replacement for a proper, in clinic consultation and skin assessment.

2

My Journey In The Skincare Industry

It all started after I attended Ryerson University in Toronto to obtain my Bachelors of Science Degree with specialization in aircraft design. Soon after, I worked at Field Aviation for aircraft modification and part design using 3D software.

When I told my boss I was quitting my job to go to aesthetic school, he laughed out loud (LOL) literally :(There are not many women working in the aerospace industry and I may be in the 0.01% to leave my engineering profession to pursue a career in the beauty industry. I liked engineering but I guess I didn't like my job. Working with metal parts was very impersonal. Against my parents' wishes, after 4 long and hard years in my aerospace bubble, I decided to go back to school to get my aesthetics diploma. After graduation I took a course specifically for lasers and worked at a laser clinic to get adequate experience.

Once I felt confident that "I knew my stuff" in-depth, I got into the laser industry with a Toronto business man, who has a masters' degree in literature from Queen's University and a Doctor who specializes in anti-aging medicine. I worked in the clinic for the first half of my career, and once I had children I worked primarily on skincare marketing and trained nurses and aestheticians on skincare theory in addition to hands on training.

Due to my tech background, I ended up taking many classes for web development at a coding school in Toronto. I then went on to study at the American Graphics Institute to improve my skills in Adobe products since I had self-taught myself the software I needed prior to attending the school. I wanted formal training to take my advertising skills to the next level.

I studied for a full year taking numerous and various classes in WordPress, HTML/CSS, UX design, SEO, video editing software, illustrating software and more. I learned how to use these programs to an advanced level and continue to take classes today to further improve my skills. I love marketing and creating content as much as I love anti-aging skincare. I will forever be a student.

Prior to completely dedicating my time to skincare marketing, "I wore many hats" meaning I was part of all aspects of the clinic's operations. I gradually took on the role of skincare marketer out of necessity. Marketing companies were not very honest making simple tasks seem complicated in order to charge more for their work and the speed at which they performed tasks really had the business at their mercy. I decided in order to grow the business, the site and advertising was something I had to specialize in, so that no marketing company could "hold the business hostage." As I took on this role as marketing director, I became a Google Adwords specialist over time. If you are interested in knowing more about my skincare marketing background, visit my website: TheSkincareMarketer.com .

3

Passion & Purpose

I am passionate about anti-aging skincare and I want to educate others on cosmetic procedures. I have always believed that clients should be educated on cosmetic treatments in detail before committing to a treatment plan. I also believe treatment providers should recommend only what people need; no more, no less.

The reality is, many people are oversold and other people are undersold, therefore, they don't get the desired results. The decision and buying process can be confusing. The solution to this confusing process is client education followed by a proper consultation and skin analysis.

Although I give you a formula at the end of this book, which serves as an activity to help you determine what type of treatments may be right for you, you need a proper consultation to solidify a treatment plan. Cosmetic treatments are elective which further makes it difficult to determine what types of treatments are right for you.

Factors to consider when deciding on a treatment plan with your physician or practitioner include your...

· Skin needs

- Desires
- Medical history
- Overall health
- Your budget
- Age
- Purpose for wanting certain treatments
- Your time commitment
- Time for healing and recovery
- Lifestyle

etc...

I stepped away from the business of skincare (client-side services) 10 years ago to focus on skincare marketing (business to business services). Now I am stepping away from B2B services to focus on skincare education.

I always felt education or knowing your services inside and out, and knowing the biology of the skin, was really the best and easiest way to market your business and dominate the industry. In other words, good marketing had to be couple with substance. It's really about just running a good business and the marketing will be easy.

I have trained nurses, aestheticians and educated doctors on laser treatments throughout my entire career. Now I want to educate **YOU**, the consumer, the client, the patient, and aestheticians/nurses on cosmetic treatments via books and courses.

Running a successful and safe clinic meant training staff according to what I believed and still believe are high standards of patient care. I created a training program and systems on how to perform treatments and protocols, early on in my career, to ensure client safety. Much like anti-aging skincare, when it comes to safety, prevention is better than correction.

Educate yourself before proceeding with any type of cosmetic procedure. There are always risks associated when having a laser treatment. These risks can be minimized with the right staff training, right technology and following through with the right pre and post aftercare.

This book will cover, what I believe, are the most effective anti-aging treatments and of course, you can participate in creating your own general treatment plan with my 3D Anti-Aging Formula™.

4

Morals And Ethics In The Cosmetic Industry

To be clear, I want to remind you that I am not a doctor or medical professional. What I failed to mention in my previous text is, aside from my technical and aesthetics background, I am also a certified TELF Teacher which means I am certified as an international English teacher. I mention this to demonstrate my passion for teaching or education in general.

Above all my credentials, I am a mother first. As much as I want to educate the client now in anti-aging skincare, I am also concerned about the morals and values in today's society that stem from vanity in this industry. We all want to look good and stay looking younger longer, however, we need boundaries or a healthier perspective on skincare and anti-aging treatments.

Skincare wasn't supposed to be solely about vanity or appearances. The skin is our largest organ. Skincare is healthcare. We need to take care of our skin from the inside-out and outside-in.

Taking care of the skin makes people feel better about themselves or confident which helps them excel in their careers and overall well-being. Many patients go into cosmetic clinics simply because they don't feel right. Looking and feeling your best from the inside-out and outside-in is good for your mental health. We just all need the right guidance and balance. Without the right guidance, balance and education, it can be harmful to our physical and mental health.

I have been in the cosmetic laser and skincare industry in general for almost 20 years. I've grown with the industry through a time when anti-aging skincare took a steep rise. Staying youthful is a BIG business and the target market keeps getting younger and younger. The direction the industry is going may be in part due to social media and this current era of social media influencers.

I believe social media influencers may be contributing to the misconception of what anti-aging really means. Influencers are asked to try different treatments yet they do not have the knowledge and background to really promote any specific type of laser treatments to their followers, let alone to the right demographic and for the right age group.

In an ideal world, anyone that has a following should take it seriously. If you are an "influencer", then you have influence over the people who choose to follow you. Take this responsibility seriously. You may not be sued for what you post, especially since the cosmetic industry already has many grey areas, however, influencers should really think twice about the impact they may have on their followers before making and releasing that skincare post.

It also really breaks my heart to see young adults at the tender age of 18 looking to start treatments such as dermal fillers to look like their favorite influencer. When young ladies have fillers, they look much older than their age. It really does not make sense to me. We all want to maintain our youth yet young girls are getting dermal fillers that make them look older.

The skincare industry is no longer about skincare. I guess the truth is, skincare treatments are literally considered cosmetic in practice, meaning they are elective and don't impose any physical health risks. We don't "need" them to be physically healthy. Cosmetic treatments though have become a stepping stone to more invasive and surgical treatments which could effect our mental health whether that be positively or negatively. Overall, we are becoming more "plastic". We are losing our individuality in the Americas on a large scale and at a "viral" pace. This pace can be in part, attributed to the "age of the influencer" where everyone wants a piece of this lucrative market. I'm not a psychologist so I'll end this section by repeating how I started.

Simply...

"I am a mother first. As much as I want to educate the client now in anti-aging skincare, I am also concerned about the morals and values in today's society that stem from vanity in this industry"

The solution is to really better educate you, the client in hopes that you care for your skin with the right intentions and guidance. This book serves to help you understand what anti-aging treatments are and skincare in general so we can all develop a healthier prospective towards cosmetic skin procedures.

5

Taking Care Of The Skin From The Inside Out

The skin is an organ which needs to be nourished. It's our largest organ and it plays an important role in the body. Our skin regulates our body temperature, disposes of toxins to a certain degree, it synthesizes vitamin D, and it is a physical barrier to the external world which works hard to keep invaders out and keep our internal body parts inside where they belong! We need to take care of our skin. It is the first barrier of protection against viruses and disease.

We all want to look younger however a facial treatment is not going to stop a virus from entering the body. I am sure you have all heard this saying and I have used it in advertising campaigns many times over:

"Take care of the skin from the inside and out" (anonymous)

Skincare is healthcare. Our skin gives us clues to what is happening on the inside of our bodies. Again, the skin is an organ and the only organ we can see. From the yellow appearance of the skin of a baby with jaundice to the growth of excessive thick facial hair on woman, the skin speaks to us and we need to listen. Our skin is a great indicator in knowing what is happening inside our bodies. If we take care of our skin on the outside, we can see these indicators more clearly. There is also a fine line as well between taking care of our skin and masking these indicators. For this reason, we need a healthy mindset when it comes to skincare since it's ultimately healthcare.

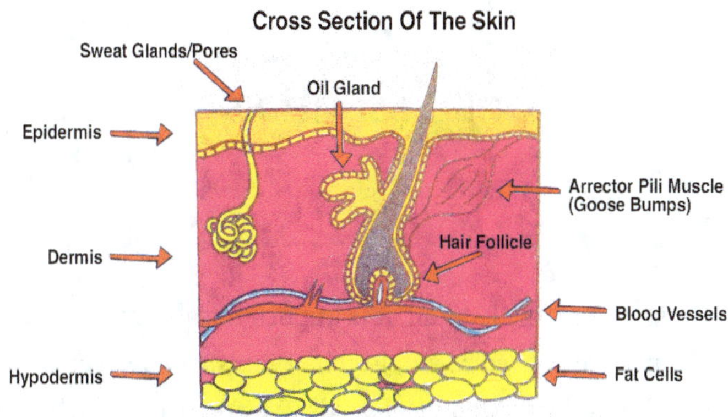

The skin has 3 main layers: the epidermis, dermis and hypodermis. It is part of a system called the integumentary system which contains our nails, sebaceous glands (oil glands), sweat glands and hair. It is responsible for regulating body temperatures, synthesizing or creating vitamin D, getting rid of toxins, balancing fluids, protecting the body from foreign invaders and more.

The skin, much like any other organ needs the right foods, vitamins, nutrients, oxygen and circulation to distribute the essentials to each and every skin cell. Let's talk a little more about the cell essentials, circulation and unhealthy addictions which not only cause pre-mature aging but effect life span and your quality of life in general.

6

Cell Essentials

Without getting into too much detail, it is important to know a little about cell biology. Life may have started as single cell organisms however today we are complex human beings with biological needs. We are made up of billions upon billions of specialized cells which all work hard to keep us alive and well. All of our cells still require the same basic needs for survival as we do as whole human beings: oxygen, food and water.

Aside: Cells also need ions for osmosis in moving what the cell needs from a higher concentration to a lower concentration (passive transport).

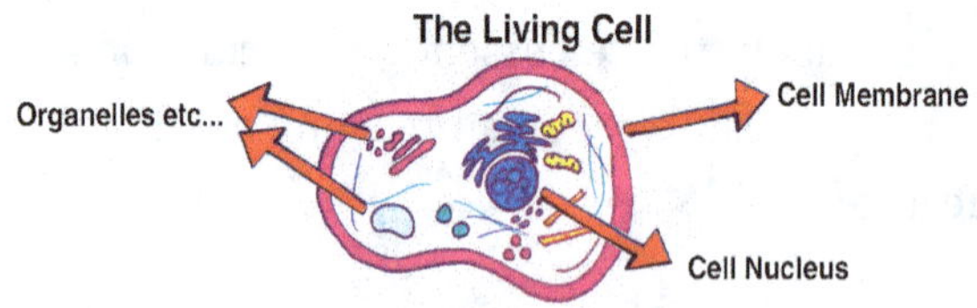

Skin cells have different forms depending on their function. Epidermal cells of the stratum corneum, which exist on the most superficial layer of the skin, are flat cells which provide a waterproof barrier for the skin. These skin cells shed, as they are designed to do. They are the farthest cells from any blood supply and don't have a blood supply in their own layer. The epidermis, has no blood vessels meaning it is avascular, therefore, it relies on the dermis (the layer below) to supply nutrients to it.

Essential vitamins and nutrients are just that, essential for cell function. When cells are not provided with proper nutrition, fluids and oxygen they die. It's that simple and if we don't give it the right nutrition and protection, we can also trigger cell mutations which cause disease.

The quality of the air we breathe, the food we eat, and water we drink affects the quality and function of each and every cell in our body whether it's a skin cell, muscle cell or immune cell.

Of course, our skin contains immune cells as well which work vigorously to keep foreign invaders out. We need to keep all of our skin cells healthy, not just the ones we can see on the surface. We need a healthy environment for our immune skin cells to do their work!

7

Blood Circulation & Staying Active

We have built in systems to ensure blood circulates throughout our body to reach each and every component of the body and cell, when we are not moving. There is an increase of blood circulation when we move.

Our extremities, such as our legs, have systems that work hard to pump blood back up to the heart. Energy is the ability to do work. Our body needs to apply energy in order to do the work of pumping blood throughout the body and to each and every cell.

Using the example of our legs, while standing, our body pumps blood back up to the heart through valves. If you ever had an injury or cut on your lower leg, you would have probably noticed that it takes a lot longer to heal then say an injury to your face. The reason being is generally, if you have two injuries, of the same magnitude, the injury that is farthest from the heart, will take longer to heal.

Going back to speaking about blood circulation with respect to anti-aging and skin health, our skin cells need blood to circulate for skin repair and rejuvenation. Cosmetic facial laser treatments are essentially designed to increase circulation to your face in order to repair and replace damaged collagen and brighten the skin. By creating controlled damage to the skin with the application of lasers, the body naturally starts the process of wound healing. This process builds collagen and elastin.

When our body's wound healing systems are activated, blood vessels are dilated to increase blood flow to the area in order to digest and repair the damaged skin. Our Basal cells, which are responsible for cell division and producing new skin cells, are activated. Fibroblasts form collagen bundles and collagen cross-linking as well as remodelling occurs. This process is only possible through the circulation of the blood.

All cosmetic lasers procedures depend on our body's natural healing process to achieve the results you are looking for: to build new collagen and tighten and/or brighten the skin.

Blood circulation is a key component to maintaining healthy skin cells and it is essential for maintaining life. We need proper blood circulation in order to deliver all the things our body needs to be healthy and heal. We should all try to make a conscious effort to be more active for our skin health and overall health.

In larger cities such as New York, many people are forced to walk since driving a car is expensive and often not the most efficient means of transport. If you are generally driving from point A to point B, then you should try to make an effort to exercise. Exercise not only stimulates blood flow, it causes the release of endorphins which are your "feel good" chemicals that make you feel happiness. Happiness also can make you look younger. We will talk more about that later!

8

Unhealthy Addictions

There are many unhealthy addictions out there however the most obvious of all bad habits is smoking. Smoking affects the appearance of the skin. Whenever I performed laser treatments on a heavy smoker during my time as a skincare/laser practitioner, I was always concerned about how the skin would not turn pink very easily during treatments that involved collagen stimulation through heat stacking.

When you add heat to an area, elevating the skin temperature to a certain degree, collagen remodeling is triggered along with an increase in blood flow, which in turn brightens the skin. Without measuring the temperature of the skin with a digital laser thermometer, a visual indication that someone is achieving results is through the appearance of erythema and inflammation of the skin. In other words, the skin should turn pink and slightly swell. These are signs that you have had an effective treatment. If the skin does not turn pink very easily, as it does not always do with those who heavily smoke, this could be a visual indication of poor circulation.

Smoking And The Skin

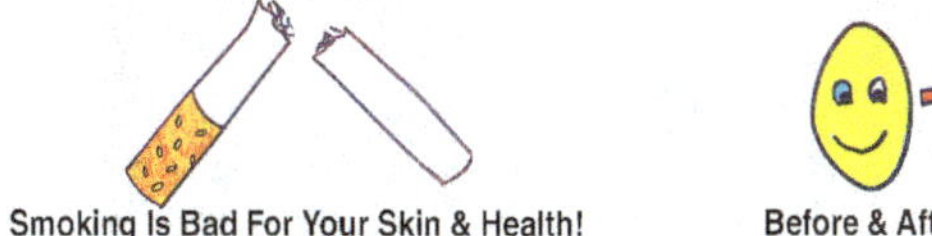

Smoking Is Bad For Your Skin & Health!   Before & After Years Of Smoking

It is a fact that smoking increases blood pressure. Smoking and second-hand smoke reduces or impairs vasodilatation. This means blood vessel walls don't dilate due to loss of elasticity in vessel walls. Smoking damages collagen in your blood vessels making them inflexible and can also create fat deposits that block blood vessels, further inhibiting blood circulation.

Blood vessels need to dilate to send blood to areas that need repair rapidly when there is bodily injury. For this reason, those who smoke, have delayed healing. Back to the first paragraph, from my experience, smokers do not turn pink very easily during laser treatments that should cause the skin to turn pink. It is much harder to treat a client for their wrinkles or for anti-aging when that person smokes as well due to delayed healing. It takes longer to see results and since the problem is one of habit, it's sort of an "up-hill battle."

In general, it is known that smoking affects the lungs ability to distribute oxygen to its cells. It destroys nutrients and reduces vitamin C absorption. I think it's pretty obvious that there are no positive health benefits to smoking. I understand smoking is an addiction which may be hard to stop, however, even cutting back can dramatically improve your health and your skin's appearance. If you decide to cut back or stop smoking for vanity reasons, that's great! Whatever makes you cut back or quit!

9

Patient Expectations

It is important to determine and understand what you want before starting a series of treatments so that you are happy with the results. There are many options out there so you need to be clear on what you want to achieve.

For example, if you go into a clinic and say you are looking for an anti-aging treatment, the consultant could recommend microneedling. Microneedling is not an aggressive treatment to get rid of any deep wrinkles. If you have wrinkles you want to get rid of, don't use the word anti-aging during your consultation. Tell the consultant that you want a corrective treatment plan to get rid of your wrinkles or you won't be given the correct recommendation.

Most people go into cosmetic clinics once they already have lines and wrinkles. If this sounds like you, then you probably do want to do some sort of skin correction before anti-aging treatments.

Correction treatments are usually more aggressive and are at shorter treatment intervals. If you want to get rid of wrinkles, you would need a series of treatments which could last 6 months to a year depending on the severity of your lines and wrinkles before committing to maintenance treatments. Skin maintenance treatments are really anti-aging treatments (prevention). One is a synonym of the other.

Cosmetic treatments are elective. When you go for a consultation, you are given recommendations, and these recommendations are based on what you are trying to achieve. You need to be clear on what you want to achieve.

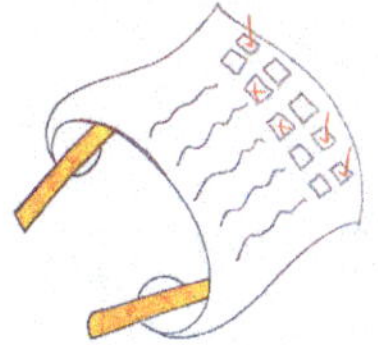

Before you go into a clinic for a consultation ask yourself:

- Do I have wrinkles I want to remove?
- Do I have pigment I want to get rid of?
- Do I have scars I want to get rid of?
- Do I have sagging skin or skin laxity I want to improve?
- Do I have acne I want to get rid of?
- Do I have recurring facial redness I want to control?
- Do I want brighter healthier looking skin?
- Do I have dark circles under my eyes I want to get rid of?
- Do I want to maintain my youth by practicing prevention or anti-aging?

If you answer yes only to the last question then you simply want anti-aging treatments. One who wants to anti-age, should commit to a skincare regimen that achieves just that, anti-aging. You don't need an aggressive series of treatments to achieve anti-aging results. You need consistent skin rejuvenation and regeneration treatments.

This is accomplished through treatments that signal the body to repair and improve the skin's appearance and strengthen collagen. Skin regeneration treatments keep the skin active and helps to rejuvenate the skin.

10

What Are Exfoliation Treatments

Before learning about exfoliation treatments, one should understand why we exfoliate our skin and what the purpose is of our outer most skin cells of the epidermis. The outer most layer of the skin is called the stratum corneum and the skin cells at its' top layer are keratinocytes.

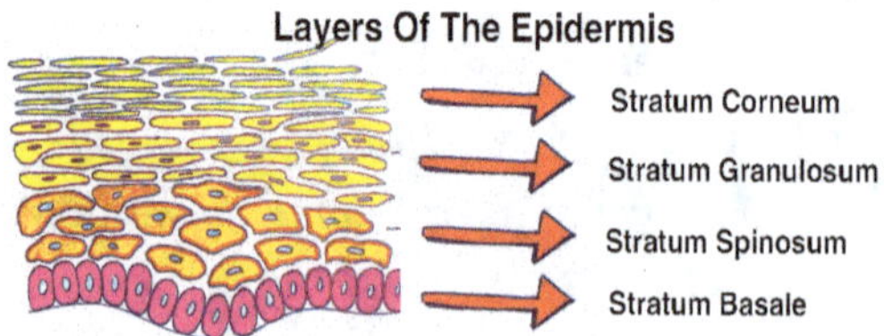

Keratinocytes really make up the majority of our epidermis. These cells are flat cells that are keratinized or for lack of biological terms "dead". Keratinized cells are specialized skin cells that are flat and have no nucleus or organelles (cell organs) like other cells. They are missing their central nervous system and organs. For lack of better terms, they are actually "dead" for a reason.

The purpose of these cells is simply to provide a water proof barrier to the skin to keep invaders out and water in. The cell wall is made of lipids or oils. These flattened cells, pilled one on top of the other, is how this barrier is formed and the reason why water and oil don't mix. Our body needs this chemistry to keep water inside our bodies. This waterproof barrier naturally sheds approximately every 30 days in the cell regeneration process to keep it healthy.

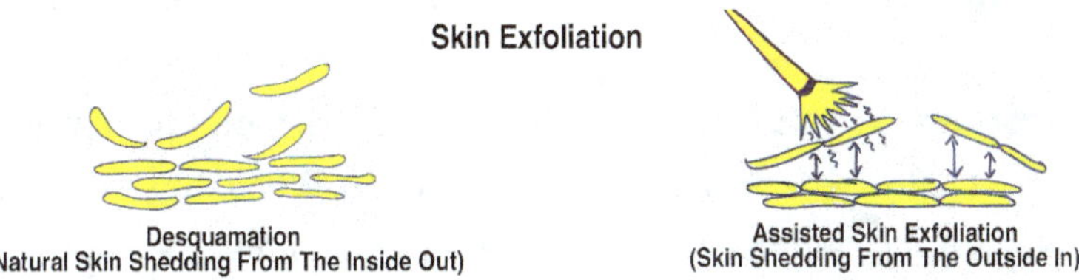

The process of natural shedding that the skin undergoes from the "inside out" is called desquamation.

The process of skin shedding through skin exfoliation is what we do to take care of our skin from the "outside in".

You may ask yourself now, if the skin naturally sheds, why do we need to exfoliate the skin?

In terms of aging, the process of skin regeneration, which occurs approximately every 30 days, slows down. When the skin exfoliates at a slower rate, this is really the onset of aging. We start to age, at the skins cellular level, approximately in our mid 20's.

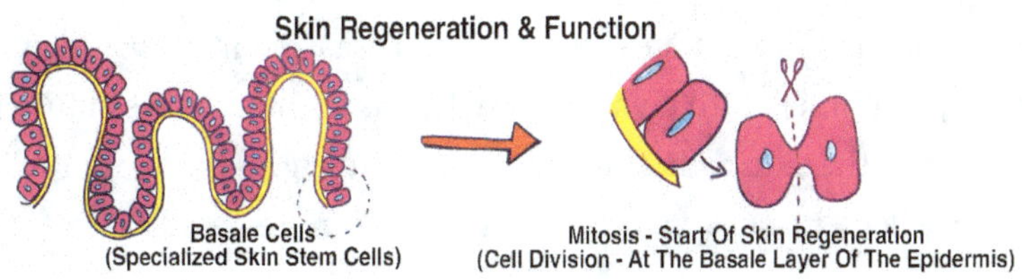

The baseline layer of the epidermis, is where basal cells exist, which undergo mitosis or cell division. These specialized stem cells divide in order to multiply to produce new skin cells every day. Skin regeneration starts with mitosis, cell division. The regeneration process is one where these basal skin cells divide in order to multiply. They then mature, specialize and move up to the surface of the skin, which is the layer we can see, and these skin cells eventually shed.

As a side note, regeneration and shedding slows down with age, however the skin can also fail to shed due to excess oil production. When the skin is too oily, the top layer of the skin fails to shed. When the skin fails to shed, infection builds up in the pores, and pimples form. This is essentially acne.

Getting back to anti-aging, by practicing skin exfoliation, we are aiding the body in maintaining the skin's youthful processes of shedding every 30 so days. Exfoliation treatments help skin cells DETACH and shed. Now that you understand shedding from the "inside out" and from the "outside in," let's summarize all of the above in one statement with the theme of anti-aging at its center:

Exfoliation treatments keep us looking younger longer by removing dead skin cells and by stimulating cellular regeneration. We are literally assisting skin shedding by helping skin cells DETACH from each other in order to shed. This makes the skin look healthy and new.

Dead skin cells can be removed from the surface either chemically or mechanically (through an acid or through physical means). Microdermabrasion is fairly straight forward to understand and makes a great example of mechanical exfoliation. During a microdermabrasion treatment, a wand with a rough surface, combined with a vacuum suction is applied to the skin, physically breaking up the skin cells at its surface. Chemical peels are more difficult to explain so let's discuss chemical peels in a bit more detail.

Skin Exfoliation With Chemical Peels

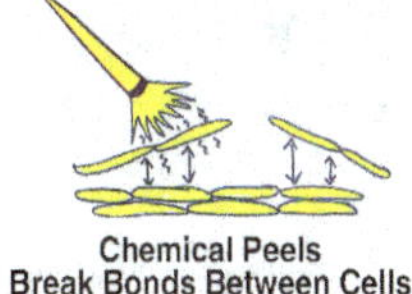

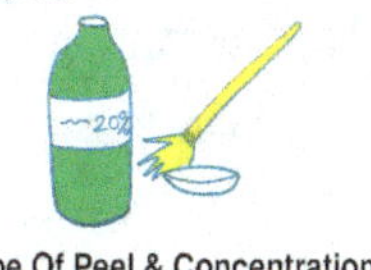

There are many types of chemical peels specially formulated for specific skin concerns and skin types. I will discuss peels in their raw or pure forms first, then talk more about new age peels which are blends of acids.

Lactic acid peels are the gentlest of all peels. They are not commonly used because they are very gentle in nature and many consumers want to see peeling or feel tingling when they get a peel. Lactic acid comes from, as the name sounds, milks. These gentle peels sooth the skin while very gently exfoliating it. They are commonly used for sensitive skin types however those with sensitive skin, tend to avoid anything with the word peel, hence why they are not commonly used anymore. If you do not have sensitive skin or have "normal" skin, you will not experience any peeling with this type of peel.

Glycolic peels are what we call alpha hydroxy acids (AHAs). Glycolic acid molecules are small in size; therefore, they can penetrate the skin easily to break apart the bonds between cells. If you simply want to keep the skin vibrant and active, use a light glycolic peel. Also, don't be disappointed if you don't have heavy peeling with a light glycolic peel. You don't need to experience heavy peeling in order to achieve anti-aging results. Usually one can expect skin flaking or dry patches for an certain period of time after a glycolic peel.

Salicylic peels differ from glycolic peels. They have larger molecules and better break down oils. Salicylic acid is a BHA or beta hydroxy acid. Salicylic peels are great for acne since they break down oils in the pores.

How are salicylic peels good for anti-aging you may ask if they are so effective for acne. Let me explain. Salicylic acid softens the skin and then easily breaks apart those keratinized skin cells at the surface of the skin. By penetrating follicles and softening keratinized skin cells, deeper peeling is provoked. You will get more of the classic conception of "skin peeling" with this type of peel.

Jessner Peels are blends of different acids. Traditional Jessner peels used to be mainly resorcinol, salicylic acid and lactic acid. Now, other chemicals or agents have been added which make them more of a chemical blend rather than a true Jessner peel. There are Jessner peels that are formulated for aging skins, pigmentation, hydration, acne, etc. Jessner peels are a great option for darker skin types with superficial pigmentation as it is difficult to get rid of pigmentation on darker skin types. I cannot really go in depth on what type of Jessner peel you may need since they are acid blends, and there are numerous blends out there. It simply isn't one acid so just make sure you educate yourself on what the ingredients are in your next Jessner peel and listen to what is recommended by your treating physician or practitioner.

In general, before trying a chemical peel or new type of peel, you may ask your treatment provider for a patch test. This would involve applying the peel to a small patch of skin, possibly a small spot on your jawline, to see if you have any adverse or allergic reactions. There are more possibilities of allergic reactions with Jessner peels since they are blends of acids. If you are using blends of acids and you have a reaction, the clinic cannot really determine the exact ingredient in the peel which caused the reaction. For this reason, a patch test may be advised for a new Jessner peel, upon review of your medical background.

In addition to the type of chemical used, there is also concentration to consider which is a major contributing factor to the intensity of the peel. The skin will peel if the concentration is strong enough. The chemistry and concentration of an acid combined, dictates the type of peeling you will achieve with any chemical peel. Salicylic peels and Jessner peels create more traditional skin peeling than glycolic acid peels or lactic acid peels. The concentration of a peel will determine the depth of penetration in addition to the peel type. Some peels can also be applied in layers further increasing its intensity.

In terms of safety, some peels need to be washed off or neutralized while others don't. Other peels rest on the skin and penetrate deeper if you add water to them. It gets complicated. Make sure you ask your practitioner for all the pre and post care instructions prior to getting a chemical peel.

My advice to you is, less is more. Start light, see how your skin reacts, then re-evaluate post every treatment to determine if the intensity should be increased or peel type changed based on your feedback. Don't rush the process. You do not need a deeper peel if you have young skin, if you do not have any skin concerns that require correction or if you do not have acne. You can actually damage your skin by over peeling or over exfoliating your skin. I have met many clients that went from clinic to clinic over exfoliating their skin which left them with acne, skin irritation and redness. Over exfoliation is real!

Over exfoliating or leaving your skin out of balance can cause photo damage to the skin from sun exposure as well. Our skin also needs to maintain a slightly acidic PH level in order to stay healthy. We need the skin's natural acidic state to protect us from the environment and free radicals in the air. Over exfoliation strips these acids away, along with our keratinized skin cells that protect us, making our skin vulnerable to the outside elements.

11

What Is A Flash Lamp

A flash lamp is a spectrum of infrared light. It is not technically a laser. A laser is a focused beam of light or one number measured in nanometers (nm). If a practitioner says their laser targets 655nm to 1064nm for example, it is not a laser. If you are told a machine targets a range of light, it is not a laser. It penetrates varying depths. It's not a focused beam of light. It doesn't mean that it doesn't work. I'm simply letting you know it's not technically a laser.

If a practitioner or doctor tells you their laser is 1550nm, in other words, one wavelength, one number, it's a true laser. True lasers have a very specific target at a specific depth of the skin. They are, **LASER FOCUSSED**!

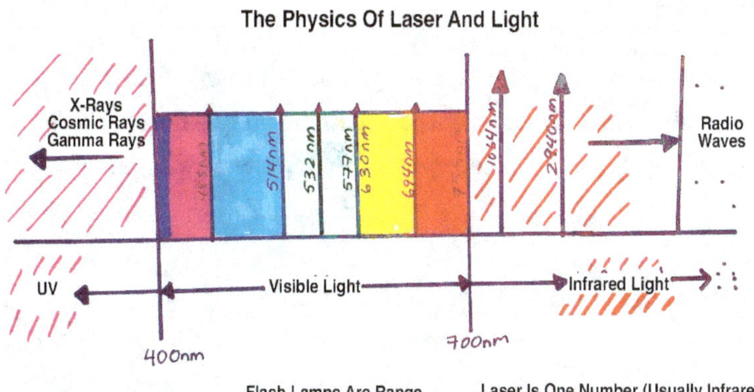

An example of a flash lamp system is IPL or photorejuvenation. Let's talk a little more about photorejuvenation, one of my favourite treatments. Photorejuvenation is often called a laser treatment however it isn't exactly a laser according to definition. Since a flash lamp is not a focussed beam of light rather a range, it penetrates varying depths and targets. Photorejuvenation is very effective for superficial pigmentation but only on fair to olive skin types. It's not an option for brown skin, tanned skin or black skin.

In general, flash lamps and lasers seek a target. They are light sources that seek a target. Once that wavelength or wavelengths find their target, they generate heat and that heat creates a desired response. Photorejuvenation targets the epidermis seen below:

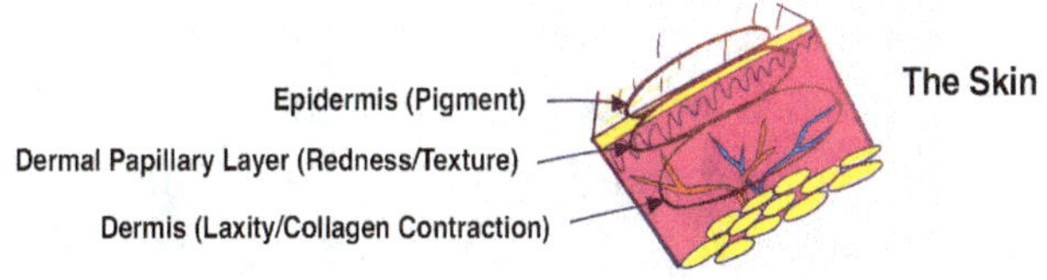

The target for photorejuvenation is red or brown dyschromia or colour in the skin. Once it finds the target, heat is generated producing a desired response. For tiny facial veins, light energy targets red in broken capillaries, generating heat to coagulate those tiny vessels.

For pigmented lesions or spots, the light seeks brown in the skin, generates heat which damages the pigmented spot. The body's natural response is to absorb the vessel or pigmented spot removing the unwanted pigment along with it.

Immediately after treatment, brown spots could appear darker. This is normal. I sometimes describe it as the appearance of coffee grinds on the skin. It actually shows that the treatment was effective and the pigment was probably superficial.

The above reaction is ideal. Superficial pigment is easy to treat. Clients love to see the spot darken and come off. Realistically though this doesn't always happen. Depending on the strength of the treatment, type of pigmentation and the depth of the pigment, one of three things could happen post treatment:

1. The spot may appear very dark and crust off (surface pigment)
2. The spot may appear darker then fade (slightly deeper)
3. The spot may simple fade (deeper pigment)

Any of the above responses are normal. It depends again on the factors I listed above (type/cause of pigment and depth of the pigment in the epidermis). Some people are disappointed if the pigment does not crust off. Really not all pigment behaves this way. If you are concerned that your pigment is very superficial and not seeing the desired results, you can always ask your provider if they can perform a patch test for your future treatment to safely be more aggressive. You can also ask for an assessment to see if there is a better treatment option for your stubborn pigment which may be the case for deeper pigment.

12

What Is A Laser

Let's talk about lasers, my favorite subject. I did describe what a laser is in the previous section but no harm in repeating it again here to reinforce what a cosmetic laser is. A laser is a focused beam of light. We measure laser light in nanometers (nm). Unlike a flash lamp, which is a spectrum of light or range, a laser is one number. One wavelength. This means that light energy is very targeted for a specific concern and depth. Here is that laser and light explanation again:

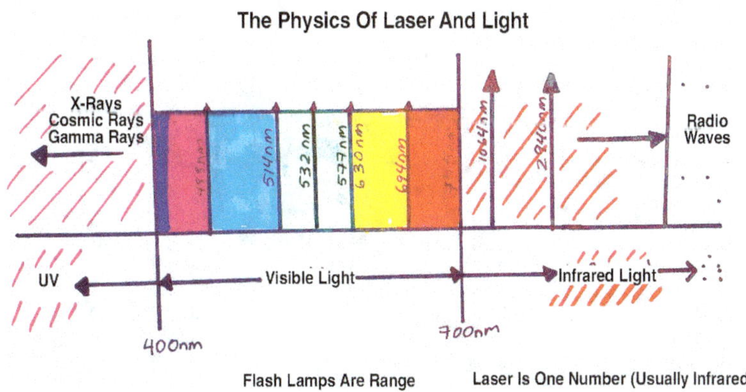

The word laser has been used interchangeably with many other technologies for skin care. The word laser, to most people, means a corrective or anti-aging treatment. I suppose there is no harm in saying "I had a laser treatment" when it isn't laser, however, technically there are many cosmetic treatments out there and laser is one of them. Lasers that go into the dermis and do not break the skin, are what we call non-invasive skin rejuvenation treatments.

Let's now go a little bit deeper. Let's talk about non-invasive laser treatments.

13

What Are Bulk Dermal Heating Collagen Treatments

The layer between the dermis and the epidermis is called the dermal papillary layer. This junction is where tiny little vessels lay. This junction is actually the start of the dermis. It is the upper most layer of the dermis. There are skin rejuvenation lasers that target this junction because these tiny vessels cause redness which are diffused rather than distinct capillaries. A term which you have probably heard, is laser facial.

Laser facials are usually 1064 nm lasers (NdYags) used for skin rejuvenation at the dermal papillary layer. Laser facials are treatments that brighten the skin, remodel collagen and help with diffused redness. It basically gives you a nice overall glow. Heat is stacked until collagen type fibers DENATURE, triggering a remodeling process which smooths out textural differences in the skin. These treatments are usually very comfortable.

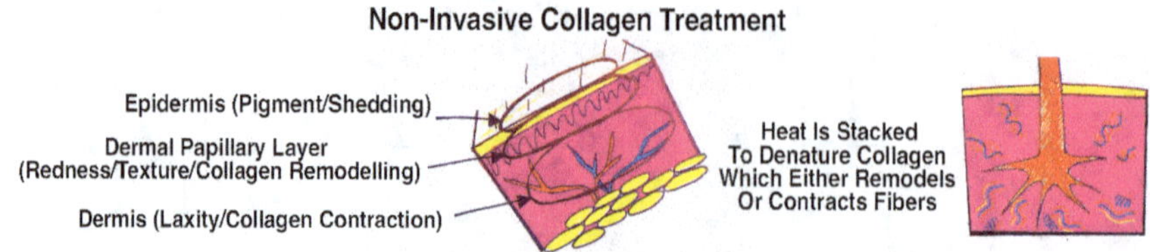

Skin tightening can also be achieved with heat stalking just at a different level of the skin. In order to tighten lax skin, we need to go deeper into the dermis. Infrared light is still used to stack heat. We want to elevate the skin temperature to the point of collagen contraction.

Laser and light treatments that work on the principle of bulk dermal heating are essentially creating a controlled response in the skin. The body will then increase blood flow and remodel collagen and elastin in the area in order for you to see the desired results which is FIRMER and more youthful skin.

We are basically stimulating the body's natural healing process, triggering fibroblasts and collagen production. This process DENATURES collagen then repairs it.

Now let's talk about non–invasive radio frequency treatments which also denature collagen.

14

What Is Radio Frequency (RF)

Radio Frequency is basically electricity. For this reason, if you have a pace maker, you should not consider RF treatment technologies. Going forward, I'll use the abbreviation for radio frequency which is RF. There are two types of RF devices: bipolar and monopolar sources. This is in reference to the flow of electricity.

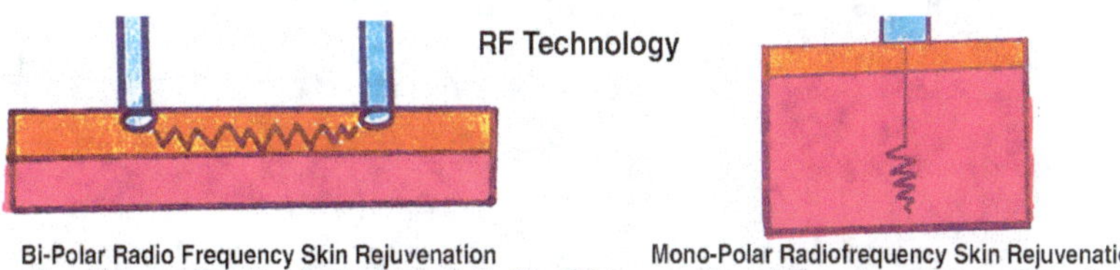

Monopolar sources are more effective in delivering energy for deep tissue building or tightening and require the patient to be the ground/escape since the flow of energy must be downward and into the skin. The energy flows through the patient and exits the patient through a pad which is applied to the client. The level of penetration is so deep that topical numbing will not make the treatment comfortable. You will feel discomfort. You can ask your doctor for pain medication and take it 30 minutes prior to treatment to ease this discomfort in order to achieve the right treatment parameters and get the best results.

Bipolar sources are more superficial since they require two electrodes at the surface of the skin. They can help to stimulate collagen on a different or more superficial level of the skin. Monopolar and bipolar sources deliver different results so again, it depends on what you are trying to achieve.

Monopolar and bipolar RF treatments denature collagen. Monopolar dermal heating with RF technology is effective for skin tightening. Heat is created in the dermis, and the body will then increase blood flow and repair the area in order for you to see the desired results which is FIRMER and more youthful skin. We are basically stimulating the body's natural healing processes, triggering fibroblasts, collagen contraction and production, similar to what we do with bulk dermal heating.

To summarize, monopolar RF sources are better for skin laxity or tightening at a deeper level of the skin. RF treatments serve to DENATURE collagen.

Next, let's will discuss collagen building with fractional lasers.

15

What Are Fractional Laser Treatments

Fractional lasers are minimally invasive treatments. A fractional laser targets a fraction of the skin. You may ask yourself, "why would I want to target only a fraction of my skin when my concerns pertain to the entire face?" Let me explain.

Scars or any textual damage of the skin, including wrinkles, and fine lines requires deeper collagen correction. If we were to remove the entire surface of the skin, which used to be the common practice 20 years ago with ablative CO_2 resurfacing laser treatments, the skins barrier would be completely exposed. These treatments that remove the entire surface of the skin, are considered 100% ablative treatments. They vaporize skin tissue. If we remove the top surface of the skin, it is up to you, the patient to care for the area. Aftercare would involve antiseptic washes to avoid infection and using some type of gel or cream to protect the skin from infection as recommended by your treating physician.

Remember the function of the skin is to protect our bodies from foreign invaders. If we remove the top surface it is up to us to protect ourselves from germs, viruses, bacteria and more. We put ourselves at risk of infection when we remove our 1st line of defense, the top layer of our epidermis.

Those who did those types of treatments in the past were at high risk of scarring. It was absolutely limited to skin types 1–3 or very fair skin individuals. The invention of fractional laser technology really changed the industry. By targeting a fraction of the skin, we are now able to penetrate deeper, we are able to treat all skin types, and we are able to reduce downtime after each treatment. Darker skin types will always have a lower safety margin in comparison to those with fair skin, however, fractional lasers allowed for skin correction of all skin types safely with the right protocols and using the right fractional laser. Let's talk about how fractional lasers actually works.

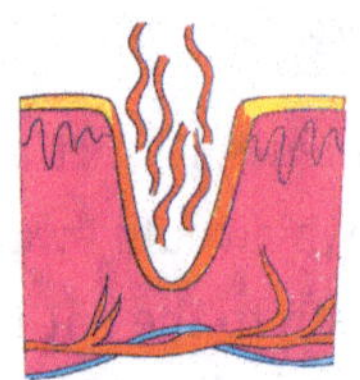

How Do Fractional Lasers Work?

Fractional Lasers Create Micro-Thermal Injury Zones In The Skin Forcing The Body To Repair And Produce New Collagen!

Fractional Lasers Are Used For Anti-Aging & Skin Correction

As I mentioned above a fractional laser targets a fraction of the skin with every treatment. Fractional lasers create thermal micro injury zones in the skin. The depth of reach can be modified by the practitioner along with the amount of coverage or spot size of each individual column. In other words, there are multiple settings a nurse, doctor, or an aesthetician can change in order to provide you the most effective correction or anti-aging treatment.

On the day of treatment, the skin is numbed for 30 minutes to 1 hour. The amount of time you need to numb the skin, depends on the strength of the numbing cream. The numbing cream is then removed and the laser is applied to the skin. Some fractional lasers require multiple passes, while others require only one pass. After treatment the skin will be pink, swollen and could feel hot. This is a normal reaction or how the skin normally acts in response to any skin trauma which is laser/heat induced. It is important not to add any more heat to the skin, not to apply any chemicals to the skin, avoid scratching the skin and to avoid sun exposure.

Once the micro thermal injury zones have healed at the surface level, it is important to remember that deeper healing is still taking place. During this second phase of healing, it is important not to do any other laser or skin treatment without consulting your practitioner or physician. Since deeper healing is taking place, it is important to realize that results from the treatment will not be evident right away. Usually any skin treatment that stimulates the process of producing new collagen growth, requires upwards of 3-6 months of healing underneath the skin which is why you should not assess the results any sooner than that time frame. Let's talk about fractional lasers for the purpose of anti-aging.

Fractional lasers used for anti-aging could be mild treatments spaced father apart. The exact spacing is really subjective for anti-aging purposes. Cosmetic treatments are elective so I can really only give you my opinion based on my experience and again, please consult your treatment provider before proceeding with any type of procedure I discuss or recommend in this book. For anti-aging, I would suggest no more than 3 light treatments a year maximum which are non-ablative. Let's discuss semi-ablative fractional lasers vs. non-ablative fractional lasers and revisit the meaning of ablative treatments.

What Are Ablative Treatments?

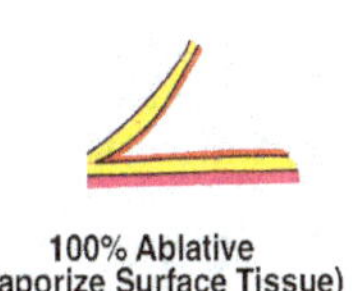

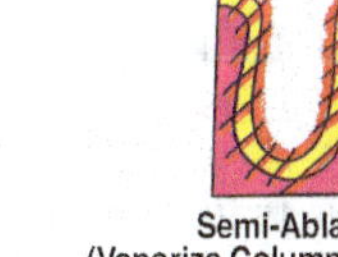

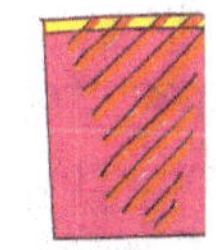

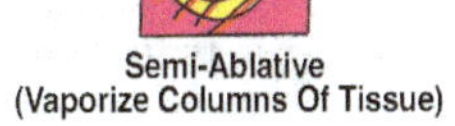

100% Ablative
(Vaporize Surface Tissue)

Semi-Ablative
(Vaporize Columns Of Tissue)

Non-Ablative
(Controlled Damage - Micro Injury Zones)

First of all, as mentioned previously, ablating the skin means vaporizing skin tissue. Ablative treatments vaporize skin tissue.

Semi-ablative fractional lasers vaporize columns of skin. Vaporizing tissue means we are removing skin tissue or "removing" columns of skin (partially vaporizing the epidermis). This is used for greater skin correction and is a form of semi-invasive skin tightening. It may not be suitable for all skin types.

Non-ablative fractional lasers are the most common type of fractional technologies used today. They damage or disrupt collagen making it ideal for anti-aging. We are not "removing" or vaporizing tissue. We are damaging it. Non-ablative means the skin is left intact. It creates a thermal injury zone without vaporizing or removing skin tissue. Non-ablative treatments are popular because they are safer for all skin types and there is low risk of infection since we are not removing columns of skin. Non-ablative fractional lasers are best for anti-aging.

Let's recap and summarize all this information above:

Non-ablative fractional laser treatments are essentially creating controlled damage to the skin. We then rely on the body's natural healing process to repair the area in order for you to see the desired results. The desired result is new collagen production leading to firmer and youthful skin. Non-ablative fractional lasers DISRUPT collagen fibers in order for your body to produce new collagen.

In conclusion, when using non-ablative fractional lasers for anti-aging, I would suggest treatments at farther intervals at lower settings than otherwise recommended by the manufacturers since those recommended settings are often for skin correction. Non-ablative fractional lasers are safer for the skin and there is little risk of skin infection assuming the treatment is performed correctly and assuming you are abiding by the aftercare instructions.

Now let's move on to talk about microneedling, another great option for anti-aging.

16

What Is Microneedling

Many people are confused when it comes to knowing the difference between fractional lasers and microneedling. The difference is huge. It's like comparing apples to oranges in terms of intensity and sophistication of technology used. First let me explain the similarities and then the differences.

Both microneedling and fractional lasers induce collagen stimulation by means of affecting a fraction of the skin each session. They both create micro injury zones. The difference is, microneedling creates injury zones, that are non-thermal meaning without the addition of heat. Without the added element of heat, we are really just puncturing the skin.

Fractional lasers can be adjusted in terms of coverage or spot size, in addition to depth, and laser intensity of course, as we are using heat to create these fractional columns. The only real setting we can adjust in microneedling is depth control. Depth is the only true parameter that can be changed because increasing the needle size could result in greater risks in terms of scarring and infection. The needle size remains consistent with professional microneedling.

Overall, by removing heat from the equation or treatment, we lose many skin benefits and precision over treating specific skin concerns. One example of the benefits of applying laser to the skin would be the coagulation affect by the laser which reduces redness. Adding heat also adds to the influx of blood flow which aids in repair and skin brightness.

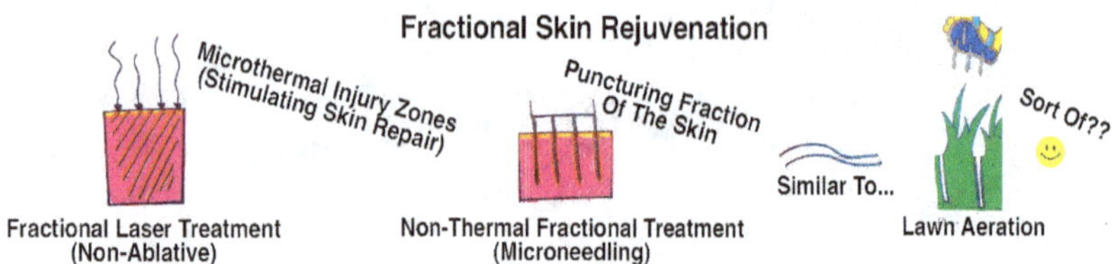

Microneedling is fairly primitive in nature. We are simply puncturing the skin with micro needles, similar to aerating your lawn. There are some people who use home microneedling systems however they are not able to penetrate very deep because it would be painful. In a cosmetic clinic, medical grade numbing is applied to the area so that the microneedles can penetrate deeper. Since we are actually puncturing the skin, there is a risk of infection. I would not recommend non-trained professionals to perform this treatment at home since proper disinfection and sanitation is required.

Many home systems don't have disposable tips and you can buy dermal rollers with varying needle sizes that would cause scarring. The cost of a microneedling treatment these days is fairly inexpensive compared to other treatment options. Personally, I don't recommend taking the risk by trying to perform a deep microneedling treatment at home. You will likely damage your skin or cause an infection.

On the day of treatment, numbing cream is applied. The microneedling wand is applied to the skin in multiple passes which could be circular, strides, or some people use a stamping method. When getting close to the eye I believe the stamping method is better and safer. It should be noted that the skin under the eye is thinner and you will see some bleeding right away if you hit a blood vessel. The depth of penetration under the eyes should be much more superficial than the rest of the face. The depth can be determined by the practitioner. This is another reason why I do not recommend this treatment at home since there are risks of complications. There are many vital blood vessels around the eyes and we definitely do not want to hit the wrong ones. As a general rule of thumb, we stay a finger width away from the eye.

The treatment takes about 30 minutes. After the treatment you will notice some pinpoint bleeding. This is normal. It will take some time for the open wounds to heal. The most superficial layer of the skin is called the stratum corneum. It takes 12 to 24 hours for the pin point openings to recover or close after a treatment. During this time, you should protect your skin by avoiding any chemicals, the sun, avoid make up and anything else that you don't want absorbed into the skin or that would cause a delay the healing process. Do not scratch the skin.

You should not feel too much heat after the treatment since we are not applying heat with microneedling, however, if you feel discomfort, cold compresses and soothing creams can help with irritation. Please make sure you consult your practitioner to ensure you are using a cream that will promote healing without adverse side effects.

Some people opt to add PRP to their microneedling treatment. PRP stands for Platelet Rich Plasma. This promotes healing and is thought to stimulate stem cell production however these claims are not proven. The results of PRP treatments are skeptical in nature however many people do say they experience greater skin improvement when adding PRP to their microneedling treatment. I have had microneedling with PRP and I have noticed some greater overall skin improvement in my skin. PRP injections are used in healthcare for tissue regeneration and healing.

Microneedling treatments are essentially creating a controlled damage to the skin. Then your body reacts and repairs the area in order for you to see the desired results. The desired result is new collagen production leading to stronger and more youthful skin.

Microneedling DISRUPTs collagen fibers in order for your body to produce new collagen. It works similarly to fractional laser treatments, to a certain degree of intensity.

17

What Is An FMR™

There are two types of injectable cosmetic treatments:

1. Dermal fillers which fill creases, lines or fill fat pockets
2. Facial muscle relaxers (FMR™) which stop the signal your brain sends to your muscle, telling it to contract, which forms lines and then wrinkles

Dermal fillers are generally used for the lower half of the face and facial muscle relaxers are mainly used for the top half of the face. Going forward I will refer to facial muscle relaxers as an FMRs™ for simplicity purposes.

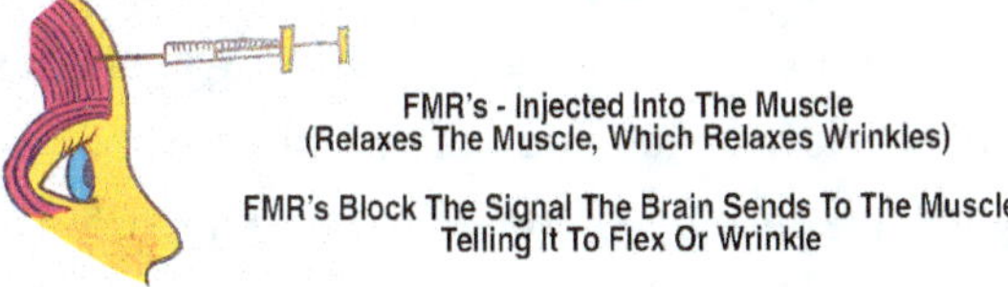

An FMR™ is typically used on the forehead, crow's feet, frown lines and bunny lines (lines on the sides of the nose). They are measured by units and injected into the muscle. What you are actually injecting is a small dosage of a toxin, a type of botulinum toxin, which is reconstituted with saline solution. Different brands may use different types of the botulinum toxin.

The number of units required really depends of the strength of the muscle. In general, frown lines usually require more units since it's a strong muscle due to repeated frowning. Men in general need more units than women since men have stronger facial muscles, genetically speaking. The more units you need, the more expensive the treatment. Some clinics charge per area while others charge per unit.

In general, an FMR™ relaxes facial muscles to treat dynamic expression lines and to prevent future non-dynamic expression lines. They prevent frown lines and prevent future wrinkles. Let's discuss the difference between dynamic and non-dynamic expression lines in greater detail.

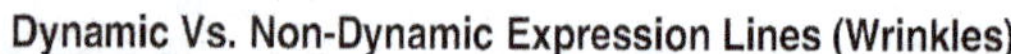

Dynamic Vs. Non-Dynamic Expression Lines (Wrinkles)

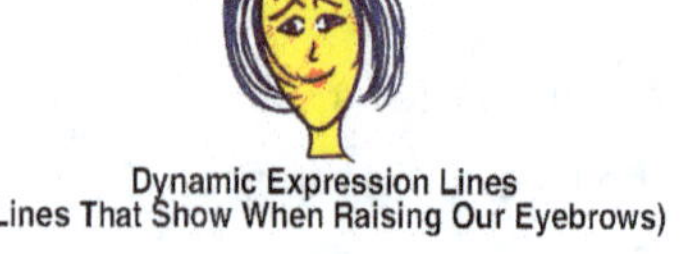
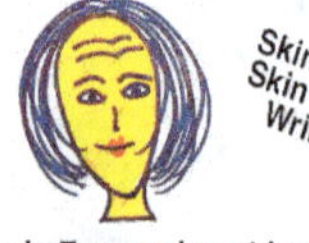

Dynamic Expression Lines
(Lines That Show When Raising Our Eyebrows)

Non-Dynamic Expressions Lines
(Lines That Show When We Are Not Showing Expression)

Dynamic expression lines are the lines which show when we smile or frown. It is the crease that forms between our muscles that we can see when we show expression. When we are not showing expression, we cannot see these lines or wrinkles. When you start seeing lines and wrinkles when you are not smiling or frowning, you have developed non-dynamic expression lines.

Non-dynamic expression lines are the lines in the skin that develop over time, when we aren't moving our facial muscles or showing expression. When we repeatedly frown or raise our eyebrows, we form creases which permanently damage the skin. This lines are what we call wrinkles. In order to get rid of wrinkles, we now need a series of correction treatments.

If you have a crease or skin wrinkle you want to get rid of it, the most effective way to do so is to have an FMR™ treatment in combination with a fractional laser treatment. This combination, will correct the damage inflicted on the skin by the muscle movement over the years. The number of treatments would vary depending on the degree of damage. Treatment intervals for FMRs™ are every 3 months and for corrective fractional laser treatments, you would need a series of consecutive treatments, spaced typically every 6-8 weeks. If you want to correct permanent creases in the skin, this combination is ideal since the FMR™ relaxes the muscle, stopping it from reinforcing the line, while the laser works to repair the skin getting rid of the wrinkle. If you have laser treatment without the FMR™, it's an uphill battle because, as we work on the skin, the line continues to be reinforced.

FMRs™ are a good option for preventing future wrinkles. Depending on your skin age and ethnicity, some people will start between the age of 25-35 for anti-aging purposes. Due to my ethnic background and considering I did have some cosmetic treatments in my late 20's, I didn't really find the need to start this treatment until I was 35. It really depends on your skin age and not always your chronological age. Many people love this treatment since the results are instant (typically seen within a week) and it makes a big overall difference in making someone look younger quickly. It's a good treatment option if you are willing to live with showing less expression on a daily basis. FMRs™ are completely different from dermal fillers.

Let's move on to talk about dermal fillers.

18

What Is A Dermal Filler

Dermal fillers are just that, products that fill the dermis or creases. I will explain how dermal fillers work however it is important to note that dermal fillers are not really anti–aging treatments. They are facial sculpting treatments or corrective treatments. Many people use fillers for fat loss in the cheeks, that may come with age or to fill creases. Others use fillers to create a more defined jawline, for lip enhancement, to create higher cheek bones, etc... Certain fillers are now even used for butt enhancement.

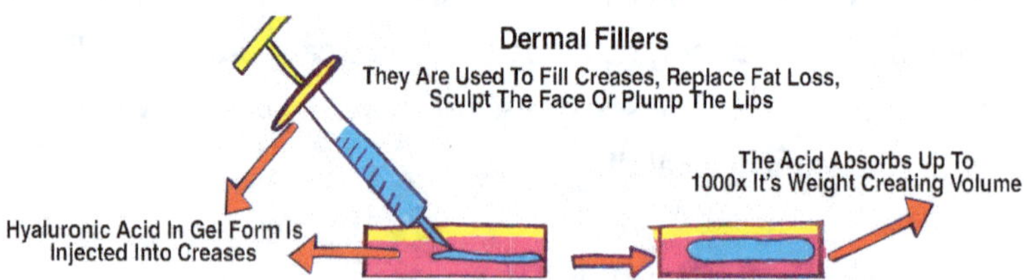

Dermal fillers are made of hyaluronic acid in the form of a gel. There are many types of fillers on the market which last for 6 months to 1 year or more depending on the size of the molecules and formulation. Hyaluronic acid is an acid we naturally have in our skin that helps us retain water and keep us lubricated. It is found primarily in the skin however naturally occurring hyaluronic acid is also required and found in the eyes and connective tissues.

Dermal fillers, are injected into creases or into an area and absorb water to create volume. It is a gel like substance that has the ability to bind to water molecules to keep us moist. When concentrated in its gel form and injected into the skin, it swells and has the ability to hold 1000x its weight in water creating volume. For this reason, it takes about a week to see the results and you should book a follow up with your physician or nurse to make sure it didn't shift or to give it time to settle.

19

What Is Pre-mature Aging

I've went over a lot of different treatment options for skin correction and anti-aging. Before we start talking about my 3D Anti-Aging Formula™, let's talk about the concept of skin age.

We have a chronological age, but we also have a skin age. Our environment, habits, diet and lifestyle all effect our skin health. Smokers, for example, could experience premature aging so if I suggest certain types of treatments and you feel you are still "aging" at the same rate, maybe you need a corrective treatment plan first or commit to a program that is for more mature skin. Just keep in mind that we can only do so much working on the outside-in. If the problem stems from the inside, it's an uphill battle.

Smoking And The Skin

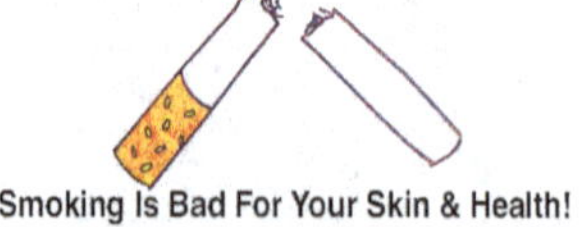

Smoking Is Bad For Your Skin & Health!

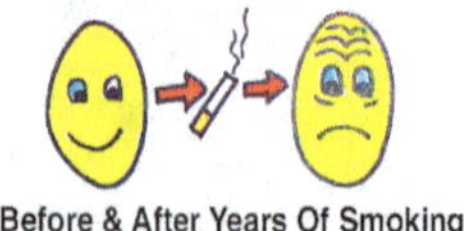

Before & After Years Of Smoking

I kept my formula general to the treatment type you need since I don't want to tell you which brand of lasers to use. I am not here to endorse any one laser company. I simply want to educate you and give you an anti-aging guideline.

Before I get started, I should mention, my anti-aging guideline states that you could start treatments around the age of 25. I'm not saying you absolutely cannot do anything before 25 but generally speaking, the skin regeneration process slowly starts to slow down at approximately age 25. Logically speaking and based on my experience, it makes sense that the approximate age we should start a clinical anti-aging plan should be around 25.

Before age 25, I suggest keeping the skin hydrated with good home care products and with the occasional facial or light peel.

Angeline's 3D Anqi-Aging Formula™

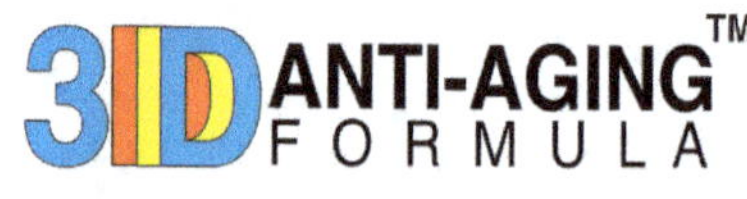

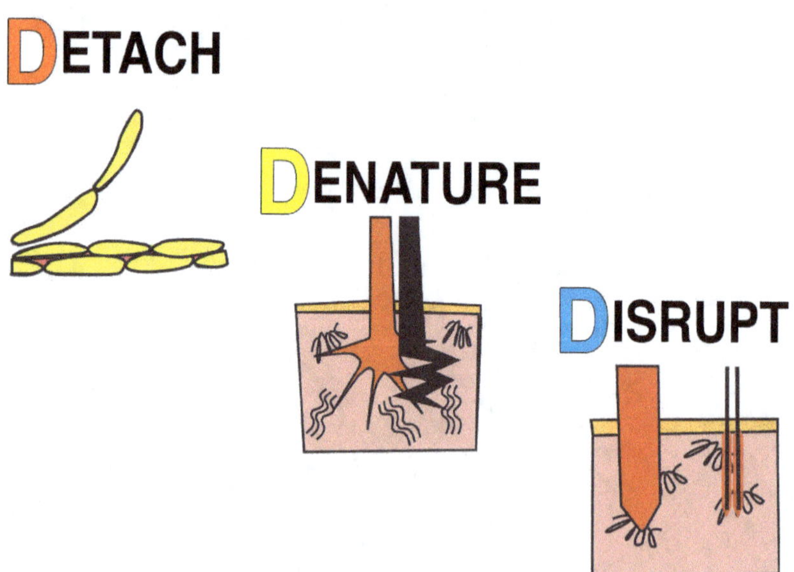

The 3–D's In My Formula Are:

DETACH DENATURE DISRUPT™

In order to achieve the best anti-aging results, I believe we should target different depths of the skin to keep it active within the course of a year. The formula is based on cosmetic procedures (the 3-D's) however you can decide if you want to add an FMR™ to your treatment plan.

I like to take-on a **"3D" approach to anti-aging** meaning I like to target different levels of the skin with different technologies to keep it healthy, active and youthful.

Before I start, I want to remind you to read the disclaimer at the beginning of this book since I am not a Physician.

Before we talk about my 3D Formula, first make the commitment of self-care. This involves you making a time commitment, financial commitment and an effort to get treatments at regular intervals.

21

STEP 1: Detach

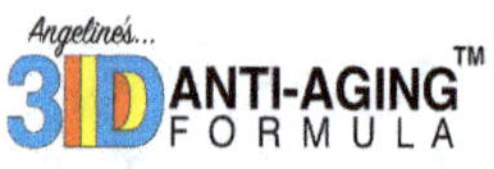

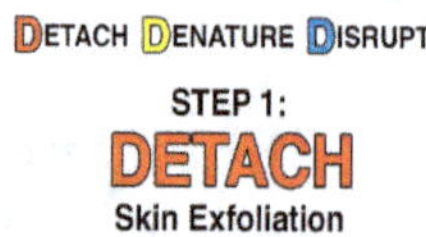

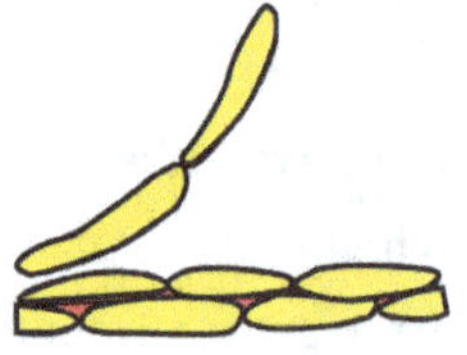

The skin's exfoliation and regeneration abilities start to degrade at approximately the age of 25. At 25, you should start to make skin exfoliation part of your treatment plan. Exfoliation treatments polish the skin to keep the epidermis rejuvenated, bright and regenerating.

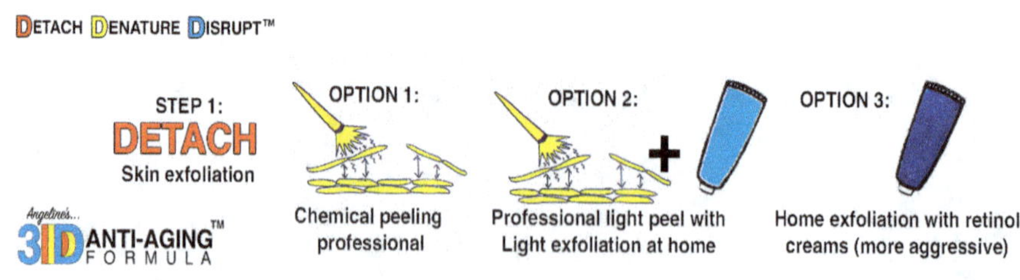

Option 1: Professional exfoliation only (25+)

If you are having professional grade peels or microdermabrasion treatments approximately every 30 to 45 days, you usually don't need anything more. You do not want to over exfoliate the skin. You do not need to use exfoliating home care products. If you are undergoing professional grade treatments, consult your physician or practitioner on what skincare products would complement your professional treatments for optimal safety.

Option 2: Light in office exfoliation coupled with light home exfoliation (30+)

If you want to use products with glycolic, lactic or salicylic acids at low concentrations, and you are going in for clinical treatments, you must discontinue use of your home care products for 7-10 days prior to treatment or you are at risk of negative side effects.

Option 3: Use of daily retinol products which are corrective in nature (approx 35+)

If you want to use high concentration or intensity exfoliation products, such as retinols, at home, you do not need to go in for clinical exfoliation treatments. Keep in mind, if you are doing any type of laser treatment, you still need to discontinue use of these products for 7-10 days prior to treatment.

Those with very thin or aged skin, may be advised not to undergo exfoliation treatments and focus on treatments which make the skin stronger and firmer, such as laser and fractional laser treatments. Prior to starting any treatment plan, please ensure you have a thorough skin analysis, by your treating physician or practitioner.

Note: the age ranges I indicate are more of a guide based on intensity of treatment, however skin age and biological age should be considered as we discussed early on in this book. Ages above are very subjective. They are an approximation based on my experience of what I think someone may require to preserve skin youth at that age.

22

STEP 2: Denature

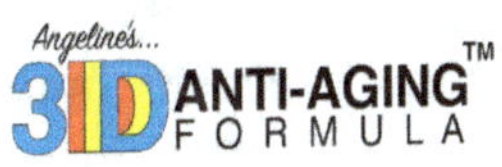

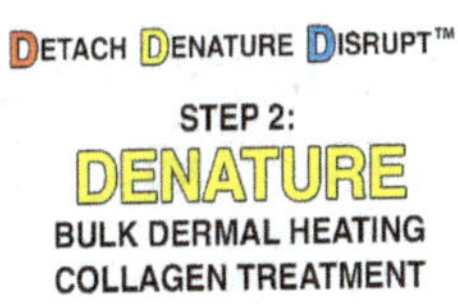

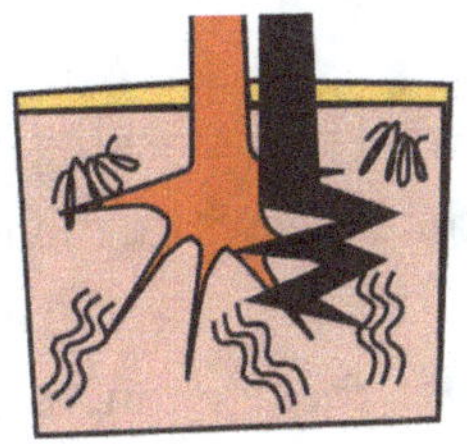

Without breaking the skin, we want to aim to remodel/reorganize collagen and elastin to strengthen and tighten the skin. By stacking heat, collagen contracts inducing new collagen, reinforcing existing bonds and signaling repair mechanisms.

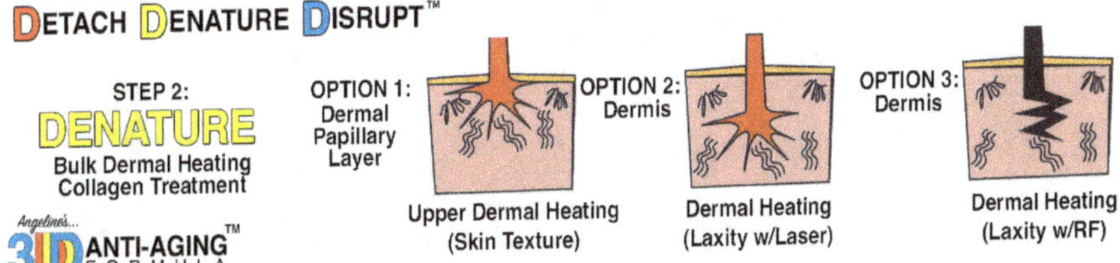

Option 1: Superficial dermal (dermal papillary) non-invasive laser treatment (25+)

You can commit to a series of laser Nd-Yag facials which target the dermal papillary layer for collagen remodeling that is more superficial.

Option 2: Deeper dermal non-invasive skin tightening with laser (30+)

You can try dermal heat stacking in the dermis with lasers which tightens lax skin.

Option 3: Deepest Dermal non-invasive skin tightening with RF technology (30+)

Dermal heat stacking can be accomplished with radio frequency as well. RF technology with a mono polar source tends to be the more expensive option.

Note: the age ranges I indicate are more of a guide based on intensity of treatment, however skin age and biological age should be considered as we discussed early on in this book. Ages above are very subjective. They are an approximation based on my experience of what I think someone may require to preserve skin youth at that age.

23

STEP 3: Disrupt

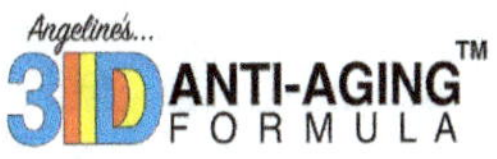

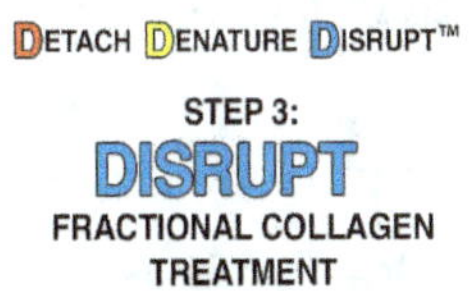

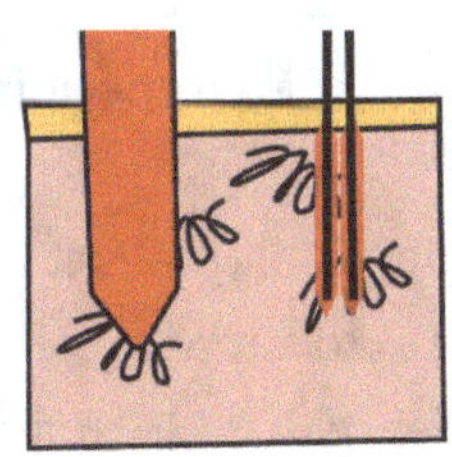

We want to physically break the collagen and elastin coils to force the body to repair the skin and produce new collagen, preventing fine lines and textual differences in the skin. This treatment triggers dermal repair, by breaking through many layers of the skin for deeper regeneration and exfoliation.

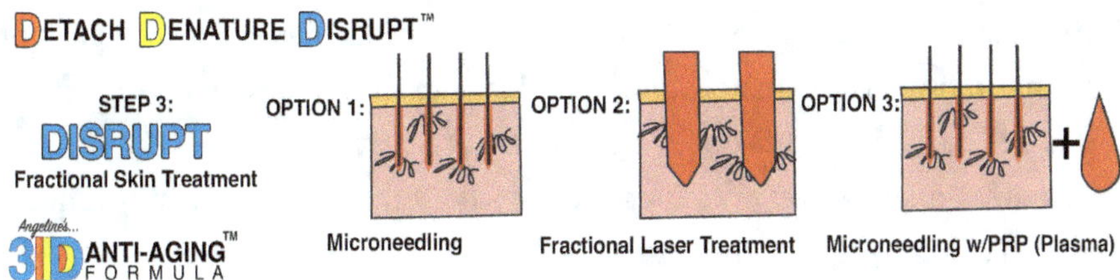

Option 1: Microneedling (25+)

This treatment is the gentlest option. Microneedling is not removing or vaporizing skin tissue (non-ablative) nor is it adding heat (non-thermal).

Option 2: Fractional laser treatment (30+)

Fractional lasers repair the skin however they can be used for anti-aging at light to moderate settings. One can have a light fractional laser treatment below 30 years of age however, usually a microneedling treatment is sufficient and a cheaper option. Fractional lasers are more expensive than straight microneedling.

Option 3: Microneedling with PRP (30+)

Adding PRP (platelet rich plasma) to microneedling, promotes healing and is said to support cell rejuvenation and repair. There is no strong clinical evidence that PRP improves the skin which is why many studies will say PRP facials are speculated to improve the skin.

PRP injections in healthcare are used to accelerate healing of injured tendons, joints, ligaments, and muscles. Adding PRP to a microneedling treatment would definitely increase the price of just a microneedling treatment alone. It's an upgraded microneedling treatment if you have the money to spend.

Note: the age ranges I indicate are more of a guide based on intensity of treatment, however skin age and biological age should be considered as we discussed early on in this book. Ages above are very subjective. They are an approximation based on my experience of what I think someone may require to preserve skin youth at that age.

24

Treatment Plan Intervals

Commit to a treatment plan that works with your lifestyle and schedule. If you can go in for an anti-aging treatment every 4 to 8 weeks, you should be on track to preserving your skin's youth or to "age more gracefully". Below are treatment plan options which serve as a guide but of course, you can always space treatments farther apart to accommodate your schedule. Some people can only make time for one treatment every change of season. There are no hard and fast rules so proceed considering the below are options.

To recap, from my experience, the best anti-aging results can be achieved through detaching, denaturing and disrupting the skin.

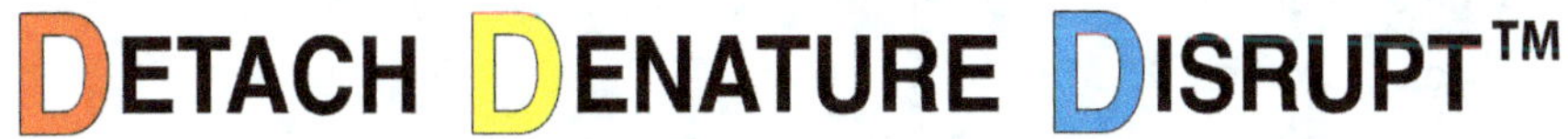

The following pages will give you options based on 4, 6 and 8 weeks intervals.

25

Treatment Plan Option 1: Every 4 Weeks

Option 1a: Every 4 Weeks (No FMRs)

- Week 1: Denature (Non-Invasive Skin Rejuvenation Treatment) + Detach (Exfoliation)
- Week 5: Disrupt (Fractional skin treatment)

Repeat...

Option 1b: Every 4 Weeks with FMR's

- Week 1: Forehead Muscle Relaxing Treatment (FMR)
- Week 5: Detach (Exfoliation)
- Week 9: Denature (Non-Invasive Skin Rejuvenation Treatment)
- Week 13: Disrupt (Fractional skin treatment)

Repeat...

26

Treatment Plan Option 2: Every 6 Weeks

Option 2a: Every 6 Weeks (No FMRs)

- Week 1: Denature (Non-Invasive Skin Rejuvenation Treatment) + Detach (Exfoliation)
- Week 7: Disrupt (Fractional skin treatment)

Repeat...

Option 2b: Every 6 Weeks With FMR's for forehead lines and wrinkles

- Week 1: Detach (Exfoliation)
- Week 7: Denature (Non-Invasive Skin Rejuvenation Treatment) + Forehead Muscle Relaxing Treatment (FMR's)
- Week 13: Disrupt (Fractional skin treatment)

Repeat...

27

Treatment Plan Option 3: Every 8 Weeks

Option 3a: Every 8 Weeks (No FMRs)

- Week 1: Denature (Non-Invasive Skin Rejuvenation Treatment) + Detach (Exfoliation)
- Week 9: Disrupt (Fractional skin treatment)

Repeat...

Option 3b: Every 8 Weeks With FMR's

- Week 1: Denature (Non-Invasive Skin Rejuvenation Treatment) + Forehead Muscle Relaxing Treatment (FMR's)
- Week 9: Disrupt (Fractional skin treatment)
- Week 17: Denature (Non-Invasive Skin Rejuvenation Treatment)
- Week 25: Disrupt (Fractional skin treatment) / FMR Same Week (Not Same Day As Fractional Laser Treatment)
- Daily: Use daily home exfoliation cream. Discontinue use of retinol or cream with acid 7-10 days prior to in clinic treatments.

Repeat...

28

Create Your Anti-Aging Guide PART 1

After reading up until this point, I assume you have a better understand of cosmetic treatments. Let me now help you apply what you have learned to come up with a treatment plan. Once you have an idea of what you may want, then you need to visit a treatment center for a consultation and solidify a treatment plan with your physician or practitioner.

Circle choices you think you may want! Dollar signs indicate approximate price scale.

1. Detach: Choose An Exfoliation Option

- Option 1: Professional exfoliation only (25+)($)
- Option 2: Light in office exfoliation coupled with light home exfoliation (30+)($$)
- Option 3: Use of daily retinol products which are corrective in nature (approximately 35+)

2. Denature: Choose A Non-Invasive Treatment

- Option 1: Superficial dermal non-invasive laser treatment (25+) ($)
- Option 2: Deeper Dermal non-invasive skin tightening with laser (30+)

($$)
- Option 3: Deepest Dermal non–invasive skin tightening with RF (30+) ($$$)

3. Disrupt: Choose A Fractional Skin Rejuvenation Procedure

- Option 1: Microneedling (25+) ($)
- Option 2: Fractional laser treatment (30+) ($$)
- Option 3: Microneedling with PRP (30+) ($$$)

29

Create Your Anti-Aging Guide PART 2

Choose Your Treatment Intervals: OPTION 1
(Feel Free To Circle Your Preference! It's Your Book!)

Option 1a: Every 4 Weeks

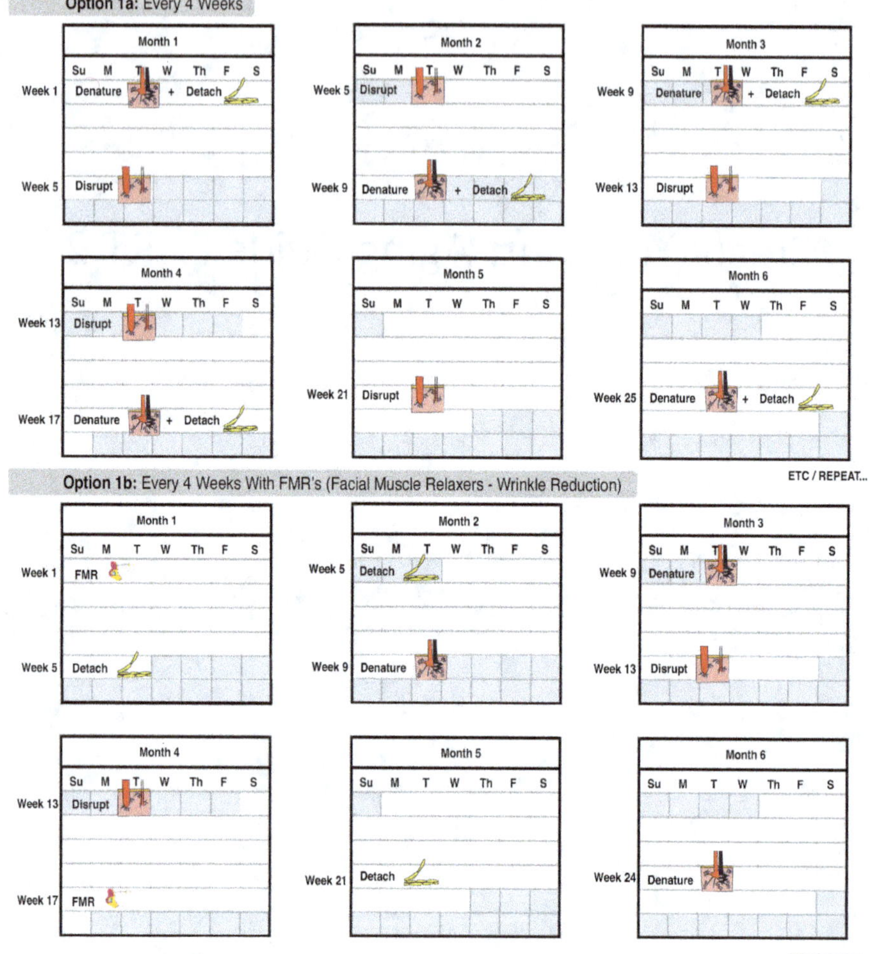

Option 1b: Every 4 Weeks With FMR's (Facial Muscle Relaxers - Wrinkle Reduction)

Choose Your Treatment Intervals: OPTION 2
(Feel Free To Circle Your Preference! It's Your Book!)

Option 2a: Every 6 Weeks

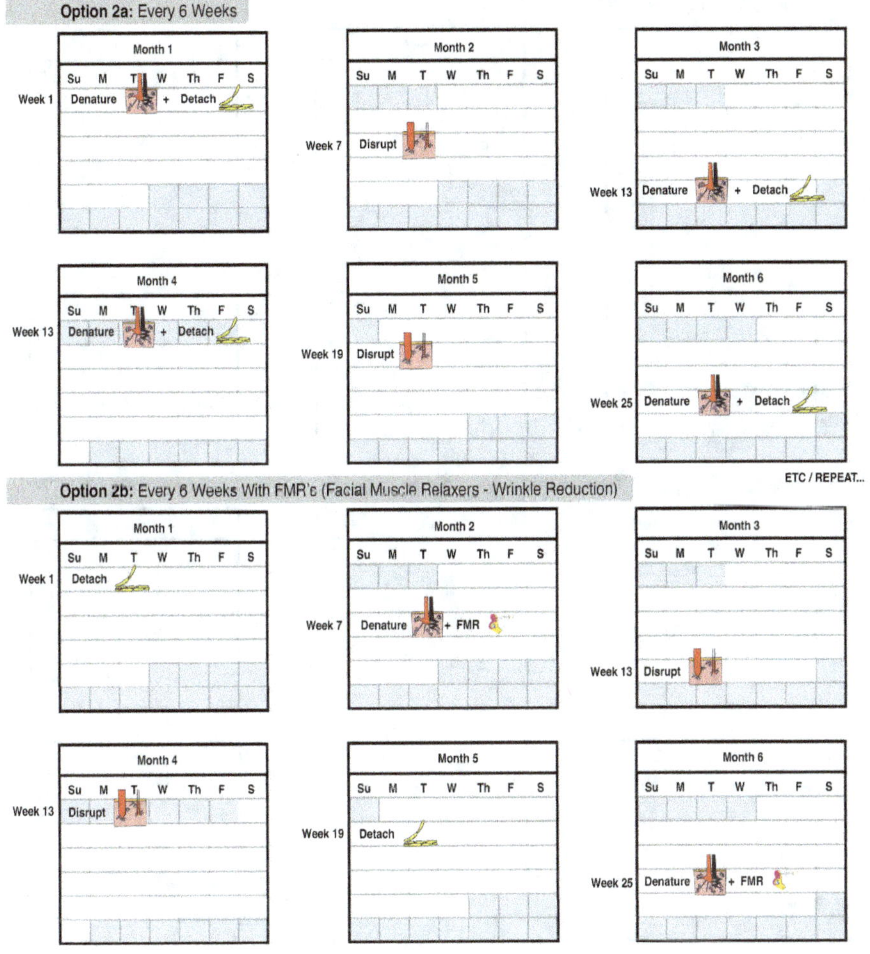

Option 2b: Every 6 Weeks With FMR's (Facial Muscle Relaxers - Wrinkle Reduction)

Choose Your Treatment Intervals: OPTION 3
(Feel Free To Circle Your Preference! It's Your Book!)

Option 3a: Every 8 Weeks

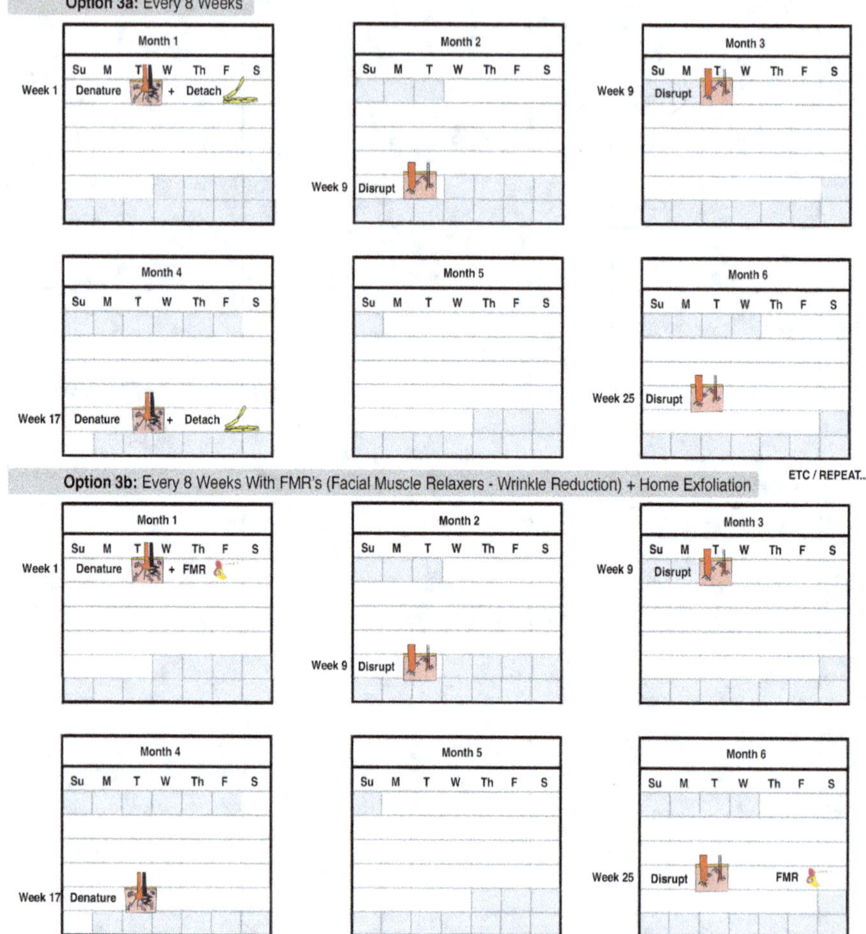

Discontue Use Of Retinols And Home Exfoliation Products 7-10 Days Prior To Treatment
On Week 25 Of Option 3b, Distrupt And FMR Treatment To Be Done The Same Week But Not Same Day

30

Complete Your Guide!

Fill in your answers from Part 1 and Part 2 here:

1. Detach:

____

2. Denature:

____

3. Disrupt:

____

4. Treatment Plan Interval:

____

Congratulations! You just completed Angeline's 3D Anti-Aging Formula™

The next step is to visit a cosmetic clinic and let them know you are ready to commit to an anti-aging treatment plan with the above in mind and they can take over from here. They can help you now by recommending the exact treatments you need which will depend mainly on the machines and cosmetic procedures the center has available, and based on your medical background. Try to find a treatment center that has a variety of lasers and procedures they can choose from.

Note: Practice Laser Safety

Normally when multiple treatments are performed on the same day, the practitioner must start with the treatment that goes deepest, then move up. Therefore, when we "Detach + Denature" on the same day, we first Denature (laser treatment first) then Detach (exfoliating the skin is more superficial). This is very important for treatment safety.

Make sure you ask your practitioner to inform you of all the pre and post care instructions for the chosen treatments. In general, after any cosmetic procedure you should avoid scratching the skin, sun exposure, exercise or inducing heat to the area. Also avoid hot water and avoid chemicals on the skin immediately after treatment and up to 7-10 days after. Please make sure you consult your physician and practitioner to avoid potential side effects.

Also, please make sure you disclose your full medical history as well, including medications you are taking, for optimal safety. Should you fail to disclose your full medical background, you put yourself at risk of negative side effects.

Should you experience any negative side effects post treatment, contact your treatment center immediately. Remember this is only a guide. Please ensure you book a proper skin consultation prior to starting any anti-aging skincare regimen.

31

My Skincare Regimen

To be honest, for the first half of my career, when I worked with clients, I did not have many treatments, except for laser hair removal and photo rejuvenation because I had freckles I wanted to get rid of. I was simply too busy working. I tend to hyper focus when I'm working and I was committed to providing excellent customer service and safety of course. I left my Aerospace Engineering bubble only to enter a new bubble in the skincare industry.

When I reached between the age of 30-35 I really felt like I needed to start prevention treatments. I was starting to get forehead lines. Due to my ethnic background, being half Asian half Italian, I really didn't need much in my earlier years.

Today I am 40 and I want to maintain healthy skin. I follow the following 6 week interval treatment plan:

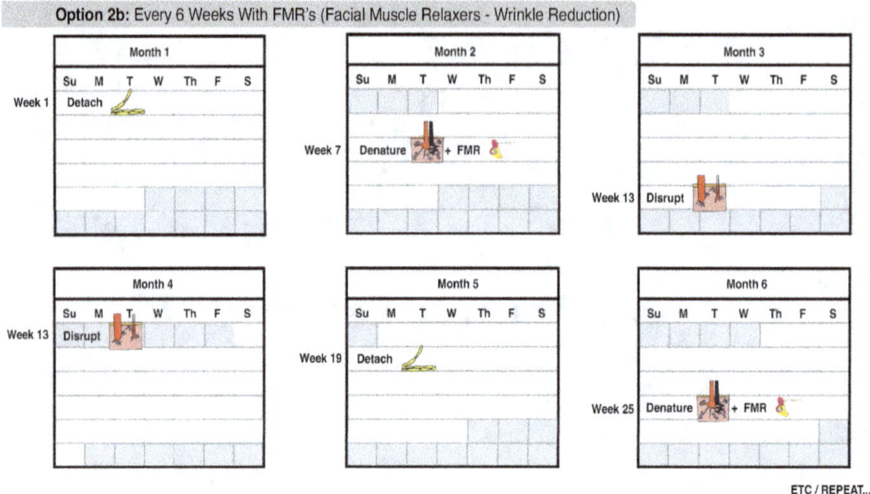

I like glycolic peels because there is no downtime and my skin feels clean and looks bright right away. I am not stuck on glycolic peels but in general I like light peels. I don't like peels that cause excessive peeling since I don't like the downtime and I don't have a lot of cell buildup that requires that heavy peeling.

I like laser facials because there is no downtime. With the right number of pulses, stimulating collagen and elastin fibers, it keeps me looking fresh and vibrant right away! It's not going to correct my skin of any textural damage spaced at these intervals but it keeps my collagen active.

I like to think of laser and exfoliation treatments as exercise for my skin. Just like a muscle gets weak and lazy, our skin starts to slow down all its life functions without the input of energy. In this case, laser energy or exfoliation treatments are the triggers which activate cells and collagen. The skin needs a stimuli and these treatments keep our skin stimulated!

I like microneedling treatments because they are minimally invasive.

I do like the effects of FMRs™. The results are relatively instant (results are visible anywhere between 3 days and 1 week). I like FMRs™ primarily for the forehead but sometimes I'll also use for my crow's feet (the lines around the eyes).

I may add one random yearly treatment just to try a new laser or experiment with different technology since it's important for me to know what's new in the industry. In general though, going back to the beginning of the book, I really like to practice what I preach which is, do what your skin needs, nothing more nothing less.

For optimal anti-aging, consistency is essential along with technology that works and experienced staff. Consistency is everything. Our habits define us. Make the commitment of self care. Commit to a skincare program that works with your budget, schedule and that is appropriate for your age and skin type.

For home care, I am not loyal to any one product line. I was never really happy with any specific product line. Since I have regular chemical peels, I do not use any products with retinols or heavy exfoliates as this would be too much exfoliation which irritates my skin. I use a moisturizing SPF product during the day and at night time I apply a nourishing serum and cream before bed. At night time the skin heals itself so I cleanse and nourish my skin before I shut off the lights. When I wake up, my skin is shiny and new!

Our bodies in general heal with sleep. I think that's common knowledge.

There are new treatments out there that actually stimulate facial muscles for the forehead and cheekbone area. Honestly, it just never ends. Just smile! It's cheaper and smiling gives you endorphins to make you feel good! Before you get sucked into the latest trend, use your common sense.

I did do some research on the effects of smiling on anti-aging in general I did find an interesting article in The New York Times which talks about smile exercises to better define the face:

"This exercise helps create a better cheekbone shape. It tightens all of your cheek muscles and helps lift the middle part of your face." [1]

This article gives recommendations for facial exercises on how to sculpt the cheeks. Could this be a way to define our cheekbones, an alternative to dermal fillers? Higher cheek bones don't help us anti-age but using or building our facial muscles does lift the skin.

[1] Times, T. N. Y. (2018c, January 10). *Exercising . . . Your Face.* The New York Times. https://www.nytimes.com/2018/01/10/well/exercising-your-facelhtm

32

Happiness & Mindset

At the risk of sounding "cheesy", from my experience, happiness should be part of everyone's anti-aging regimen. I believe when we are happy we naturally glow and radiate beauty. To me being beautiful isn't just about physical traits. It's a state of being. It is all encompassing in who we are as people. I believe when we are happy, healthy, confident, and ourselves, our personality shines and we become "more beautiful."

One thing that is apparent is that over the years, more and more people are taking anti-depressants and many people who are lonely, who can afford treatments, come in simply for the experience or for companionship. They just want to feel good. We all want to look younger but many people, of all ages, go into cosmetic clinics because they simply don't feel right. It's not even physical, it's mental.

A clinic can provide the best services and treatments possible for patients, however, we can only do so much when the problem is deeper. I am not a psychologist or certified therapist however, when someone came in for a treatment in the past, and if I could make them feel good about themselves and smile, I noticed they automatically looked better. This is what I see anyway (the eye of the beholder). In my opinion, when people smile, they look better and younger.

Although the problem may not be entirely physical for some people, the body and mind are one. I believe, how we feel and how we look changes who we are and how we act. Sometimes we become what we look and feel like, so make sure what you look like, coincides with what you feel like or want to feel like.

Thanks for listening and I hope you enjoyed this book.

Bye for now!

Angeline

33

Conclusion

To those who took the time to read this entire book,

I know I mixed a bit of my own moral and ethics at the beginning and end of this book. The opinions and guidelines I expressed is skin knowledge I have from my schooling, research throughout the years and references cited at the end of this book. Really this book is just my experience and an expression of who I am as a person as well or my perspective of what is a healthy mindset towards skincare.

In order to have a healthy mindset in regards to skincare, we have to educate ourselves on the skin and all these cosmetic treatments available so we can then make educated choices. If you filled out "Angeline's 3D Anti-Aging Formula™", remember to discuss the exact treatment plan with your treatment center or doctor. Consider recommendations they may have during your consultation outside of this guideline as well.

I hope you learned something from this book and thank you for your time.

Kindest Regards,

Angeline

Feel free to follow me on my social media accounts!

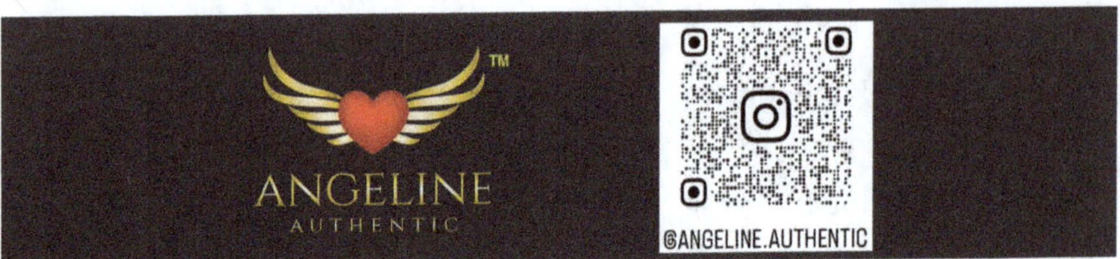

34

References

Times, T. N. Y. (2018, January 10). *Exercising . . . Your Face.* The New York Times. https://www.nytimes.com/2018/01/10/well/exercising-your-face.html

Grujičić, R., MD. (2022, December 5). *Papillary layer of dermis.* Kenhub. https://www.kenhub.com/en/library/anatomy/papillary-layer-of-dermis

Kirsch, M. B. K. S. (1998, October 1). *Ultrastructure of Collagen Thermally Denatured by Microsecond Domain Pulsed Carbon Dioxide Laser.* Dermatology | JAMA Dermatology | JAMA Network. https://jamanetwork.com/journals/jama dermatology/fullarticle/189445

Laughter Helps Blood Vessels Function Better. (n.d.). ScienceDaily. *Laughter Helps Blood Vessels Function Better.* (n.d.-b). ScienceDaily. https://www.sciencedaily. com/releases/2005/03/050310100458.htm

Fried, I. (1998, February 12). *Electric current stimulates laughter.* Nature. https://www.nature.com/articles/35536?error=cookies_not_supported& code=8e9f2ac8-7786-41e0-bb5b-99f62f6ec89a

Vergin, J. (2019, April 11). *It's possible to train our "humor muscle."* dw.com. https://www.dw.com/en/you-can-actually-train-your-humor-muscle/a-48

278350

Morrill, H. (2021, November 2). *Charting: A Brief History of Anti-Aging.* Harper's BAZAAR. https://www.harpersbazaar.com/beauty/skin-care/a14980/history-of-anti-aging/

The difference between natural desquamation and exfoliation: What it means for your skin. (2018, December 19). Griffin+Row. https://www.griffinandrow.com/education/skin-biology/skin-physiology/difference-natural-desquamation-exfoliation-means-skin/

Reduce Fine Lines & Wrinkles | Laser Skin Revitalization. (2018, October 15). Cynosure. https://www.cynosure.com/treatments/fine-lines-and-wrinkles/

Pigmented Lesions. (2021, August 22). Cutera Aesthetic Solutions. https://www.cutera.com/face-and-body-solutions/pigmented-lesions/

Thermage | Skin Tightening Treatment. (n.d.). https://www.thermage.com/

Fraxel | Skin Resurfacing Treatment. (n.d.). https://www.fraxel.com/

NCBI - WWW Diagnostic. (n.d.). https://www.ncbi.nlm.nih.gov/pmc/articles/PMC6603175/

Facial Volume Loss | JUVÉDERM®. (n.d.). https://www.juvederm.com/volume-loss

Allergan Aesthetics | An AbbVie Company. (n.d.). Allergan Aesthetics. https://www.allerganaesthetics.com/

Wikipedia contributors. (2022, June 13). *Keratinocyte.* Wikipedia. https://en.wikipedia.org/wiki/Keratinocyte

Just a moment. . . (n.d.). https://www.osmosis.org/notes/Skin_Structures

NCBI - WWW Blocked Diagnostic. (n.d.-b). https://www.ncbi.nlm.nih.gov/pmc/articles/PMC7399440/

Just a moment. . . (n.d.-c). https://www.researchgate.net/publication/259696785_Laser_fractional_photothermolysis_of_the_skin_Numerical_simulation_of_microthermal_zones

xeo®. (2021, December 8). Cutera Aesthetic Solutions. https://www.cutera.com/solutions/xeo/

Times, T. N. Y. (2018c, January 10). *Exercising . . . Your Face.* The New York Times. https://www.nytimes.com/2018/01/10/well/exercising-your-face.html

www.ingramcontent.com/pod-product-compliance
Lightning Source LLC
Chambersburg PA
CBHW061257250726

48653CB00002B/676